About the Authors

Alyesha Proctor is an advanced paramedic practitioner and independent prescriber working in general practice. Alyesha is also a Fellow of the Higher Education Academy and previously worked as a senior lecturer in Paramedic Science at the University of the West of England. Alyesha received a National Institute for Health and Care Research Clinical Doctoral Research Fellowship to develop an intervention to support paramedics to safely assess and manage children with minor head injury. She has a passion for all aspects of prehospital care and her particular interests include the clinical decision-making processes that occur in the out-of-hospital setting, the interfaces between primary, secondary and ambulance care, the evaluation of prehospital interventions to reduce avoidable conveyance and the impact of multidisciplinary teams in primary care. Alyesha has a keen interest in sexual health and contraception, as increasingly primary care practitioners are expected to have generalist knowledge on a range of sexual health and contraception issues. Alyesha has also completed the Faculty of Sexual and Reproductive Health Diploma.

Hettie Lean has had an extensive career as a practice nurse and nurse practitioner in a range of settings, including primary, secondary and community care within the NHS and voluntary sector. For 12 years, she worked as a nurse/nurse manager for Brook, a national charity offering clinic and outreach services for young people, as well as training for professionals across the UK. Hettie is a senior lecturer in sexual health at the University of the West of England and a Fellow of the Higher Education Academy. In 2015 she became a member of the Faculty of Sexual and Reproductive Healthcare, the Royal College of Obstetricians and Gynaecologists – being one of the first nurses to achieve the Diploma of the Faculty of Sexual and Reproductive Healthcare and Faculty Registered Trainer status. She continues to engage in practice as a nurse in community contraception and sexual health clinics.

■ Contributor

Emma Painter is a matron and senior safeguarding nurse at Unity Sexual Health, University Hospitals Bristol and Weston NHS Foundation Trust. She holds a BSc (Hons) Psychology, and a BSc (Hons) Adult Nursing. Emma

About the Authors

started working in sexual health in 2008. She has had experience as a sexual offences nurse examiner, working at The Bridge, Sexual Assault Referral Centre in Bristol. In 2022, Emma completed her psychodynamic psychotherapy training with Severnside Institute for Psychotherapy, and is registered with the British Psychotherapy Council.

How This Book Works

This book, written by clinicians actively involved in the clinical management of sexual health, is part of the *Primary Care Essentials* series, which aims to target the increased range of clinicians now working in primary care.

Each chapter contains signposting to resources including relevant research, guidelines for practice, suggestions for further reading and case studies to aid reflection. The following symbols are used to highlight specific practice points.

 Important points to remember.

 Risk mitigation and management in decision making.

 Ethical considerations.

 Further reading is provided where it may be useful to read more about a subject. The title of the publication is given with a citation. The full reference can be found in the further reading list.

 Cross-references. Directions to other pages in the book which may be useful.

 Safeguarding responsibilities.

How This Book Works

 Health promotion.

■ A Note on Terminology

We have chosen to use the words 'woman/women' to represent people with female anatomy and the words 'man/men' to represent people with male anatomy. In so doing, we do not seek to exclude people who do not identify according to the anatomy of their body, but use the terms that exist in the clinical guidance for this topic area. In Chapter 1: Communication, we have identified the importance of using inclusive language when working with individuals who identify as non-binary and transgender.

■ Disclaimer

The details in this book are presented for information purposes only. Practitioners should always work to local protocols and within their own level of governance and experience. Though information on examination and prescribing is provided in this book, you should not examine someone unless competent to do so or prescribe without expertise or further training.

Your employer may not provide the same brand of contraceptive mentioned in the text and therefore any brands shown are for example purposes only. The information contained herein with regard to brand names does not constitute endorsement or recommendation.

■ List of Abbreviations

2WW – two-week wait

AIDS – acquired immunodeficiency syndrome

ARV – antiretroviral

AYPH – Association for Young People's Health

BASHH – British Association for Sexual Health and HIV

BBV – blood-borne virus

BHIVA – British HIV Association

BMI – body mass index

BMS – British Menopause Society

BNF – British National Formulary

BV – bacterial vaginosis

CBT – cognitive behavioural therapy

CHC – combined hormonal contraception

COCP – combined oral contraceptive pill

CSE – child sexual exploitation

Cu-IUD – copper intrauterine device

CVD – cardiovascular disease

EC – emergency contraception

ED – emergency department

EE – ethinylestradiol

FBC – full blood count

FGM – female genital mutilation

FPA – Family Planning Association

FSH – follicle-stimulating hormone

FSRH – Faculty of Sexual and Reproductive Healthcare

GBL – gamma-butyrolactone

GHB – gamma-hydroxybutyrate

HCP – healthcare professional

HIV – human immunodeficiency virus

HRT – hormone replacement therapy

IDSVA – independent domestic and sexual violence advisor

IM – intramuscular

IMB – intermenstrual bleeding

IUC – intrauterine contraceptive

IU/l – international units per litre

IUS – intrauterine system

IV – intravenous

LAM – lactational amenorrhea

LARC – long-acting reversible contraceptive

LGBTQ+ – lesbian, gay, bisexual, transgender, queer/questioning, plus many other terms used to define sexual orientation and gender identity (such as non-binary or asexual)

LH – luteinising hormone
LMP – last menstrual period
LNG – levonorgestrel
LNG-IUS – levonorgestrel intrauterine system
MSM – men who have sex with men
NAAT – nucleic acid amplification test
NHS – National Health Service
NICE – National Institute for Health and Care Excellence
NSAID – non-steroidal anti-inflammatory drug
NSPCC – National Society for the Prevention of Cruelty to Children
PCOS – polycystic ovary syndrome
PEP – post-exposure prophylaxis
PHE – Public Health England
PID – pelvic inflammatory disease
PIL – patient information leaflet
PMDD – premenstrual dysphoric disorder
PMS – premenstrual syndrome
POI – premature ovarian insufficiency
POP – progestogen-only pill
PrEP – pre-exposure prophylaxis
SARC – Sexual Assault Referral Centre
SNRI – serotonin and norepinephrine reuptake inhibitor
SSRI – selective serotonin reuptake inhibitor
STI – sexually transmitted infection
TFT – thyroid function test
TV – *Trichomonas vaginalis*
TVUSS – transvaginal ultrasound scan
UKMEC – United Kingdom Medical Eligibility Criteria for Contraceptive Use
UPA – ulipristal acetate
UPSI – unprotected sexual intercourse

USS – ultrasound scan
UTI – urinary tract infection
VTE – venous thromboembolism
WHI – Women's Health Initiative
WHO – World Health Organization

Introduction

Many practitioners working in primary care are expected to have generalist knowledge of sexual health issues and contraceptive queries. However, they may have very little experience of managing these types of presentations. This handbook provides a quick reference guide for practitioners working in primary care using contemporary, evidence-informed guidance, including that provided by the Faculty of Sexual and Reproductive Healthcare (FSRH). The aim is to enable practitioners to gain confidence in the assessment and management of care for patients presenting with sexual health issues and contraceptive queries. A variety of topics are covered, including the importance of communication when working with patients who present with sexual health issues, a recap of male and female sexual and reproductive anatomy and physiology, methods of contraception including emergency contraception and legal and ethical considerations, the menstrual cycle and complications related to it, the menopause, sexually transmitted infections and safeguarding.

No such handbook could claim to cover the topic of sexual health and contraception in its entirety. We therefore refer to a range of courses in the book that we feel are appropriate and conform to UK clinical standards.

CHAPTER 1

Communication

■ Introduction

Many people are extremely anxious or embarrassed when discussing sexual health issues such as sexually transmitted infections (STIs), contraceptive methods or sexual response difficulties. Factors such as stigma, fear and negative attitudes from the practitioner can prevent or inhibit people from discussing sexual health concerns with healthcare providers (Bauer et al., 2016; Gore-Gorszewska, 2020). The age, gender identity and experience of the practitioner can also affect how comfortable a patient will feel when discussing sexual health concerns (Hinchliff and Gott, 2011). It is therefore essential that healthcare professionals (HCPs) communicate in a way that puts people at ease.

■ Self-Awareness When Discussing Sexual Health Issues

Box 1.1 lists some negative feelings which may arise when discussing sexual health issues.

Box 1.1

Embarrassment; shame; fear; anxiety; disappointment; sadness; impatience; frustration; inadequacy; humiliation; mortification; pride; nervousness; inhibition; reticence; reserve; caution; ineptness; anger; judgement; prejudice; disgust; confusion

Before thinking about the emotions that patients might be feeling when discussing intimate and sensitive details about sexual behaviour, we need to address the range of feelings that we, ourselves, might be feeling or mirroring during a consultation. This includes examining how our own attitudes and values might have an impact on how the individual feels and how much they are prepared to disclose to us. For example, our body language and tone of voice can give subtle clues about discomfort or disapproval when issues such as unusual sexual behaviours and abortion are being discussed.

Sexual Health and Contraception

> **Reflective activity**
>
> Circle the words in Box 1.1 that you have felt, or might feel, when talking about intimate matters with patients. This activity is best undertaken with a trusted colleague, particularly if you are able to discuss real-life scenarios and ways of responding that may help to put people at ease.

 However experienced we are, there can still be times when a patient describes a situation that we find difficult or when we feel we did not respond in a helpful way. Clinical supervision or reflecting with a mentor or colleague can start with the question: 'I'm not sure I handled this well, how might you have handled the situation?'

■ Communication Skills That Help to Put Patients at Ease

The words listed in Box 1.1 illustrate the sometimes uncomfortable nature of discussing sexual health concerns. The following list offers some suggestions of communication skills that can be utilised to help put our patients at ease.

- Adopting a warm and friendly manner when greeting a patient.
- Using appropriate body language, such as maintaining eye contact (if culturally acceptable), having an open posture, smiling and nodding to show you are listening and to encourage them to continue, and having minimal engagement with the computer.
- Using open questions initially, followed by an exploration of initial concerns and more closed questions as the consultation continues.
- Explaining the confidential nature of the consultation and the rationale for asking certain questions.
- Using language that is sexually explicit, clear, understandable and words with which you are both comfortable.

 Examples of specific wording are offered further on in this chapter in Box 1.2.

■ Environmental Factors That Can Improve the Quality of Communication About Sexual Health

- A welcoming, comfortable physical environment.
- Clear display of literature that stresses confidentiality.

CHAPTER 1 • Communication

- Clinic administration procedures which are designed to ensure confidentiality is maintained – consider, for example, visibility of clinic files and lists.
- Consultations take place in private, sound-proofed rooms.
- Students and observers are present only with the patient's consent – this should be obtained before the patient enters the room.
- A chaperone is offered for any intimate examination.
- Accommodation, where possible, of requests for specific clinician gender on the basis of culture, religion or personal preference with pathways to other services in place to support patients whose preferences cannot be accommodated.
- All advertising of the clinic, including websites and leaflets (in other languages where possible), explains the role of the clinic and what to expect during a consultation.

An e-learning module on chaperones and consent is available via e-learning for healthcare (NHS, 2022a).

■ Addressing Language Challenges in Communication

All healthcare settings should have policies in place to address the communication needs of patients whose first language is not English, people with hearing or learning difficulties and people who cannot read.

Some resources to aid communication where there are language challenges are:

- sign language interpreters
- foreign language interpreters
- access to telephone interpretation services
- use of communication aids, including websites
- working with local support organisations
- dedicated clinic times for patients with communication problems.

■ Communication to Facilitate Cultural Safety

A fundamental principle of communication in healthcare is the promotion of cultural safety. Cultural safety in healthcare refers to the experience of the recipient of care. Comparable to clinical safety, it allows the patient to feel safe in their interactions with HCPs and promotes opportunities for people to take control over their health. This can be particularly important for those who experience disempowerment in their everyday lives due to issues such as stereotyping, racism, homophobia and transphobia.

Communication is a vital component of enabling cultural safety for working with any group of people who share common characteristics, such as language, social practices, or values and attitudes. The concept of 'cultural safety' was developed in New Zealand to address barriers and health inequalities faced by indigenous populations. Cultural safety aims to address power imbalances in healthcare interactions by acknowledging historical, social and systemic barriers (Allen-Leap et al., 2022). While the use of this approach is predominantly promoted within First Nations communities, the principles are applicable to a UK context (Lokugamage et al., 2023). The fundamental aim of cultural safety is:

> '...based on the premise that culturally safe actions by the health professional will lead to more positive experiences and improved health outcomes for patients. Implementing cultural safety principles into practice will require any health professional to engage in a process of transforming their practice through identifying culturally unsafe behaviours and being willing to engage in discomforting and challenging critical reflection on your own values, attitudes and behaviours' (Best, 2017).

Best (2017) highlights the following principles to address cultural safety:

- Reflective practice: recognising conscious and unconscious biases that may affect your provider–patient interaction. Continuously reflect on how your own cultural identity can have an impact on your professional practice.
- Consider power differences: understanding the importance and impact of power and privilege, in both your role as a health professional and your individual characteristics (culture, age, sexuality etc.). Ask yourself 'are my actions empowering or disempowering my patients?'.
- Engagement and discourse: practising empathetic, respectful and open patient-centred care, for example culturally appropriate body language.
- Decolonisation: being mindful of the historical and ongoing effects of colonialisation and intergenerational trauma.
- Consider exploring cultural safety training to enhance your practice.

■ Raising Sexual Health Issues in Everyday Practice

An opportunistic approach to addressing sexual health issues in non-specialist sexual health settings, such as primary care, can help identify sexual health issues that might otherwise remain overlooked or unaddressed. For this to be effective, HCPs can be encouraged to think broadly about sexual health issues, rather than limiting questions of a sexual health nature to consultations where the primary focus is contraception or concerns about STIs.

The PLISSIT model (Annon, 1976) is a framework developed to help HCPs introduce sex into a clinical conversation and then offer appropriate counselling, treatment and referral. The acronym signifies four levels of intervention.

- **P**ermission
- **L**imited **I**nformation
- **S**pecific **S**uggestions
- **I**ntensive **T**herapy.

In developing this model, Jack Annon (1976) suggested that most people can resolve sexual problems if they are given:

- permission to be sexual, to desire sexual activity, and to discuss sexuality
- limited information about relevant sexual matters
- specific suggestions about how they might address their sexual problems
- appropriate intervention or referral.

The framework was developed further by nurse educators Bridget Taylor and Sally Davis (2007) and renamed the Ex-PLISSIT model. This extended version reinforces the importance of explicit permission giving (Box 1.2) and review as core features of each stage of interaction with patients.

The Ex-PLISSIT model encourages the HCP to consider their own level of knowledge and comfort as well as the circumstances and comfort of the patient. The HCP might decide to bypass the stages of giving information and suggestions if they do not have the expertise in these areas. This could mean referring to specialist services such as psychosexual therapy, relationship counselling, urology or gynaecology.

The Ex-PLISSIT model focuses on reflection and review for both the patient and the practitioner.

> **Box 1.2** Questions to help raise discussion on sexual health issues (permission giving questions)

- 'People with [a specific condition/on this medication] often experience sexual difficulties, such as loss of desire or problems with enjoyment. How have you been affected?'
- 'Many people are concerned about how this condition and/or treatment might affect their sexuality. What is your experience?'
- 'How has your health affected you as a couple? Has it affected your sexual relationship? Would you like to talk about this?'
- 'Do you think you may have sex when travelling overseas? Have you thought about how you can stay safe/minimise risk?'
- 'Have you previously been tested for any STIs or HIV?'

See *Discussing Sexual Health with Your Patients* (CDC, 2019) for more information.

Sexual Health and Contraception

■ Taking a Sexual History

The initial contact with a patient can be particularly important in terms of taking an accurate sexual history and making it easier for a patient to access services in the future. If you develop a good rapport, the patient will find it easier to return for subsequent visits or enquiries about sexual health concerns.

Whether the focus of the consultation is identifying STIs, providing contraception, pregnancy counselling or any other routine or acute sexual health matter, taking a sexual history will often help to identify underlying concerns that patients have. Many are too shy to raise their concerns and will only discuss their sexual health concerns if the HCP asks relevant questions (Panay, 2018; Ports et al., 2014). Where HCPs engage in open conversations about sexuality and sexual health, patients are more likely to open up and talk about concerns such as sexual dysfunction or potential STIs that might otherwise go undiagnosed, causing delayed treatments (Bauer et al., 2016; Nash et al., 2015).

Reflective activity

How comfortable are you with using or hearing the following words/phrases/behaviours?

Anal sex; oral sex; sex toys; fisting; group sex; chemsex; open relationships; polyamorous relationships; (mutual) masturbation; erectile dysfunction; premature ejaculation; orgasm; female sexual response; S&M; strangulation; pornography...

Consider asking colleagues to tell you 'the most awkward question I've ever been asked was...' and discuss with them appropriate responses and ways of dealing with our own discomfort in such situations.

Key points for taking a sexual history

- Initiate the consultation with a confidentiality statement and the rationale for asking intimate questions, followed by open questions, an exploration of the patient's initial concerns and then more closed questions as the consultation continues (see Boxes 1.3 and 1.4).
- Take a brief, core sexual history to establish if someone might be at risk of STIs (see Box 1.4); this can be followed up with a more detailed history if test results are positive.
- Explain that questions about risk taking, which some patients might find offensive (such as injecting drug use), are asked of everyone.
- Be aware of the signs of anxiety and distress from the patient, including non-verbal cues.
- Avoid assuming that an older patient is no longer sexually active due to their age and therefore thinking it inappropriate to ask (Ezhova et al., 2020).
- Use clear, understandable, sexually explicit language (see Boxes 1.4 and 1.5).

CHAPTER 1 · Communication

Examples of wording of questions

It is easy to stray into asking questions about a patient's medical, obstetric, contraceptive or family history, especially if this is more familiar and comfortable for you. The questions in Box 1.4 will help you stay on course and focus specifically on taking a core sexual history. These questions provide examples of the words you might use to address the list of topics that should be covered when taking a sexual history.

Box 1.3   Initiating a conversation about STI risk

'Hello, my name is [...]. Welcome. What brings you here today? How can I help you?'

- 'I'm going to ask you some questions to establish whether you are at risk of any sexually transmitted infections, such as chlamydia. These are questions I ask all patients in order to assess accurately their risk of STIs. Please don't take it personally and be assured that this information is kept in strict confidence unless you or someone else is being hurt or is in danger.'
- 'Do you have any questions before we get started?'
- 'Have you ever been tested for STIs before? If so, what were these and when was this? Did this include testing for blood-borne viruses (BBVs) such as HIV?'
- 'Have you had any recent symptoms such as pain when you pass urine, discharge from vagina/penis, lumps or bumps in the genital area?'

Box 1.4   Key questions when taking a core sexual history

As early as possible in the conversation, the following set of questions need to be asked in the order that they are listed.

1. 'When did you last have sexual contact?'
2. 'Who was that with? For example, a regular partner or one-off encounter?'
3. 'What is the gender of that person?'
4. 'Was that vaginal, oral or anal sex or masturbation? This helps us decide on which tests to take and where from.'
5. 'Was a condom used?'
6. 'Was this sex you consented to or were happy to have?' (For young people, ask the age of the contact.)
7. 'When did you last have sexual contact with someone else?'

If the answer to question 7 reveals that there has been another sexual contact within the previous 3 months, repeat the set of questions from point 1.

 Additional questions are required to assess the risk of BBVs such as HIV, syphilis, hepatitis B and C. See Box 1.5.

7

Sexual Health and Contraception

 UK National Guideline for Consultations Requiring Sexual History Taking: Clinical Effectiveness Group British Association for Sexual Health and HIV (Brook et al., 2020).

Multiple partners

Sometimes when you ask the question about whether the person has had sexual contact with anyone else, it becomes obvious that it might be useful to ask the following question.

'How many partners (approximately) have you had sexual contact with in the last three months?'

When multiple partners are disclosed, for example, more than three in the last three months, it is acceptable to summarise the number of partners and type of sexual activity, rather than specific details about each contact.

Box 1.5 Key questions when assessing the risk of BBVs

These questions can be initiated by explaining 'I am going to ask some questions to help assess your risk of BBVs such as HIV, syphilis and hepatitis B and C'.

Question	Rationale
(To a man) 'Have you ever had sex with a man or with a transgender woman?' *(To a woman)* 'Have you or your sexual contacts had sex with a man who has sex with men or transgender women?'	Men who have sex with men (MSM) and transgender women have been shown to be at higher risk of BBV acquisition. To identify the need for hepatitis B, C and HIV testing and hepatitis A and B vaccination and offer risk reduction advice.
'Have you or your sexual contacts ever used needles to inject drugs?'	To identify the need to test for hepatitis B, hepatitis C and HIV, also the need for hepatitis A and B vaccination.
'Have you ever paid for sex or been paid for sex?'	Sex workers face a significantly increased risk of BBVs (hepatitis B, C, syphilis and HIV).
'Have you had sex with a partner who is from a country with a high HIV prevalence such as sub-Saharan Africa?'	To help identify a higher risk of HIV.

CHAPTER 1 • Communication

 For further information on HIV, see pp. 95–99 in Chapter 7: Sexually Transmitted Infections.

Responding to Concerns Around Sexual Difficulties

It is essential that HCPs are confident about initiating and engaging in conversations when patients may have concerns related to sexual difficulties such as those listed below. This should include knowing when and how to make onward referrals, using appropriate terminology, to other practitioners and agencies such as psychosexual health, dermatology, gynaecology and urology.

Common sexual difficulties in women
- Reduced sexual desire
- Difficulties achieving orgasm
- Dyspareunia (painful sex)
- Vaginismus (involuntary tightening of vaginal muscles making penetration painful/difficult)
- Symptoms associated with the menopause
- Functional difficulty due to, for example, disability, surgery, genital conditions or illness.

Common sexual difficulties in men
- Erectile dysfunction – can be a symptom of cardiac disease (always investigate further or refer on)
- Premature ejaculation
- Delayed ejaculation
- Reduced sexual desire
- Functional difficulty due to, for example, disability, surgery, genital conditions or illness.

- The British Association of Urological Surgeons (2023) website has a section called 'Patients: 'I think I might have...' offering information and guidance on men's health issues, including those listed above.
- *The Relate Guide to Sexual Intimacy* (Campbell, 2015).
- *Sexual Wellbeing For All* (2023) provides information and resources for people experiencing a variety of sexual difficulties and problems.

Communication with Specific Groups

The latest version of the British Association for Sexual Health and HIV (BASHH) guideline for consultations requiring sexual history taking (Brook et al., 2020) offers new recommendations for communicating around female genital mutilation (FGM) and with users of chemsex. The guideline also suggests considerations for working with transgender (and non-binary) individuals.

Communication around female genital mutilation

Questions enquiring whether previous FGM has been performed should be routinely included for all cis-gender women and those assigned as female at birth (Brook et al., 2020). The language we use around FGM requires sensitivity. Some women find the word 'mutilation' offensive or difficult to hear and may prefer the term 'female circumcision'. This is controversial as this term can be associated with 'male circumcision', minimising the harm and mortality associated with FGM. You should try to mirror your patient's language. If the woman does not know what you mean when asking about FGM, you could try the following question: 'Have you ever had any operations or been cut on your vulva/genitals?'.

Information about types of FGM and protocol to follow when women have experienced FGM is covered on pp. 114–115 in Chapter 8: Safeguarding.

The following principles should be embedded in any initial conversation when a woman has disclosed FGM.

- Give the message that the individual can come back to you at another time if they wish.
- Give a very clear explanation that FGM is illegal and that the law can be used to help the family avoid FGM if/when they have daughters or family members at risk.
- Offer support, for example counselling, NHS FGM specialist clinics, Statement Opposing FGM leaflet which is available online with a variety of translations (Gov.UK, 2021).
- Do not assume that families from practising communities will want their girls and women to undergo FGM.

Communication with users of chemsex

A useful definition of the term 'chemsex' is provided by McCall et al. (2015).

> '"Chemsex" is used in the United Kingdom to describe intentional sex under the influence of psychoactive drugs, mostly among men who have sex with men. It refers particularly to the use of mephedrone, γ-hydroxybutyrate (GHB), γ-butyrolactone (GBL), and crystallised methamphetamine. These drugs are often used in combination to facilitate sexual sessions lasting several hours or days with multiple sexual partners.'

Advice and practical tips for professionals engaging in supportive roles for people using chemsex are offered by the Change Grow Live charity (2022) and include the following.

- Supporting someone who is using chemsex drugs should begin with an open, honest conversation. It is important to explore each person's situation, including what drugs they are taking, how often, and their physical health, mental health, and social circumstances.

CHAPTER 1 • Communication

- Everyone's situation will be different, and the support they need will vary. If someone is experiencing issues with their mental health, you could direct them to local mental health support services. If they identify as LGBTQ+, you could direct them to specialist LGBTQ+ services.

 Further reading, including advice and guidance on chemsex and a harm reduction approach for crystal meth, mephedrone and GHB/GBL, can be found on the Change Grow Live website (2022).

Communication with individuals who identify as transgender and non-binary

This section offers some practical suggestions to be aware of and to adopt when holding conversations with people who identify as transgender and non-binary. It is adapted from the BASHH (2019a) document.

- Ask every patient how they identify their gender and which pronouns they use as part of routine enquiry. Always use their chosen name, pronoun and/or title.
- Ask 'what gender are your partners?' as part of routine enquiry with all patients rather than 'do you have male or female partners?'.
- Misgendering someone (for example, using 'she' instead of 'he') can be highly distressing to trans people. If this happens, apologise immediately and acknowledge your mistake and then move on with the consultation.
- Ask about a patient's preferred language when it comes to their body and genitals and mirror their language in the consultation.
- Not all trans people will have had, or want to have, gender-affirming treatments such as hormonal medication or genital surgery.
- Avoid assumptions about their anatomy and how they have sex. Using models or diagrams may be more helpful than 'anatomically correct' terminology.
- Explain that you are asking so that you can understand what specific sexual health tests they may need.
- Remember that trans individuals experience higher rates of violence, domestic abuse, sexual abuse and harassment than cis-gender individuals. They may also be more likely to be involved with commercial sex work, and to misuse drugs and alcohol. Sensitive questioning about this should be part of routine enquiry with all patients.
- Cervical screening is recommended for everyone with a cervix but may be psychologically or physically challenging for trans men and non-binary people. Consider and offer opportunistic cervical smears if appropriate to trans men and non-binary people, which may need additional labelling to avoid rejection by local laboratories. Encourage participation with breast, bowel and abdominal aortic aneurysm (AAA) screening programmes, remembering that individuals may be missed from automatic recalls following a change of gender marker on primary care records.

Sexual Health and Contraception

Work within your competence. If specific advice or knowledge is necessary (for example, managing genital postoperative complications), seek advice from your local surgeons and specialist gender services.

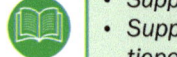
- *Transgender Health: A practitioner's guide to binary and non-binary trans patient care* (Vincent, 2018).
- *Supporting Trans Patients: A quick guide for GPs* (Transactual, 2021).
- *Supporting Transgender Adults: A guide for primary care practitioners* (The Clare Project, 2021).
- *LGBT Health Hub* (Royal College of General Practitioners Learning, 2023).

■ Summary

This chapter has addressed communication in relation to sexual health for HCPs in primary care. As in any setting, the golden rule is to listen. This means checking our assumptions and the way our values and attitudes might affect the way we respond in consultations when addressing sexual health issues. It also means considering an individual person's needs within the wider context of their lives to enable sensitive, safe and appropriate services.

CASE STUDY

Instead of a traditional case study, I have chosen to offer this short film (10 minutes). It captures the essence of what makes a difference for people identifying as trans, non-binary and queer. The accessibility of healthcare services for this patient group is discussed from 6 minutes in. It was created by Off the Record (Bristol) and Educational Action Challenging Homophobia (EACH).

▶ Search: *What is Gender? (Inspiring Equality in Education)*

CHAPTER 2

Anatomy and Physiology – A Recap

■ Introduction

In order to be able to differentiate between what is normal and what requires attention, HCPs working in primary care need to have a basic understanding of the anatomy and physiology of the female and male reproductive systems and the influence of hormones. In this chapter, we outline some basic information about anatomy and physiology in relation to the most common sexual health presentations in primary care.

■ The Female Reproductive System

The female reproductive system comprises the pelvic organs: two ovaries, two fallopian tubes, the uterus, cervix and external genitalia. This, and some surrounding anatomy, is depicted in Figure 2.1.

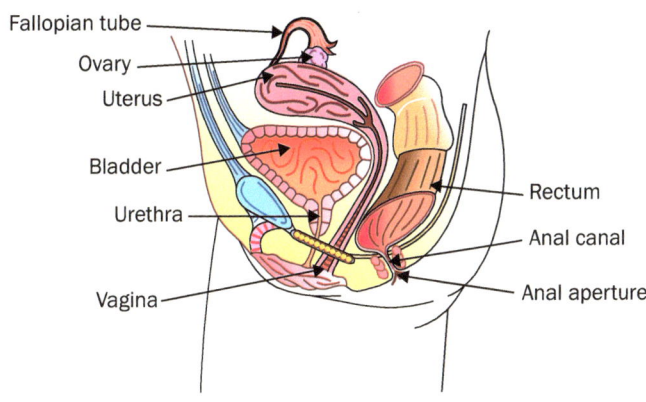

Figure 2.1 Female reproductive system.

13

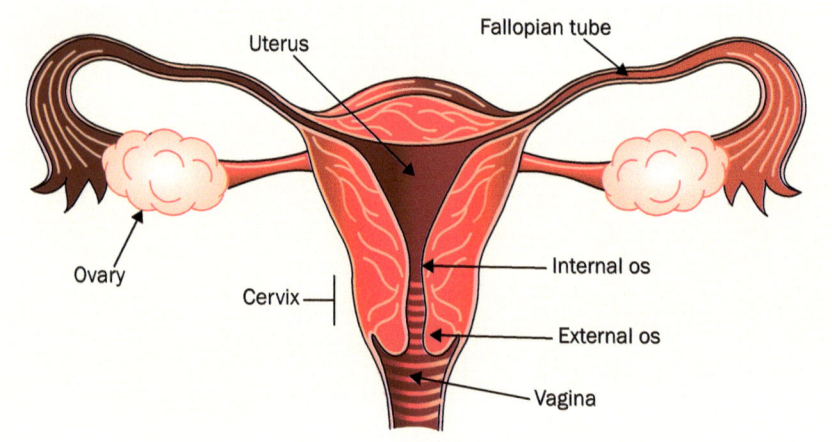

Figure 2.2 Anatomy related to the menstrual cycle.

The menstrual cycle

When women present with symptoms related to menstruation, a starting point is understanding the anatomy and physiology of the menstrual cycle. Figure 2.2 names the main anatomical features involved in the menstrual cycle.

The menstrual cycle is regulated by the complex interactions of the following hormones: luteinising hormone (LH), follicle-stimulating hormone (FSH), oestrogen and progesterone. There are three phases to the menstrual cycle: follicular (before the egg is released), ovulatory (release of egg) and luteal (following egg release). A typical cycle occurs every 21–35 days with an average cycle lasting 28 days. This is depicted in Figure 2.3.

 For more information see Chapter 5: Menstrual-Related Complications (pp. 55–69).

Pregnancy – calculating gestation

When engaging with pregnant women, there may be times when identifying a woman's individual menstrual cycle can help with determining how advanced a pregnancy is or the most likely time a baby will be born if the pregnancy goes to full term (38–42 weeks). Gestational age is measured from the first day of the last menstrual period (LMP) to the current date, with an assumption that conception would have occurred halfway through an average 28-day cycle. The estimated date on which a baby is likely to be born at term can be calculated by adding nine months and seven days to the first day of the LMP or using a

CHAPTER 2 • Anatomy and Physiology – A Recap

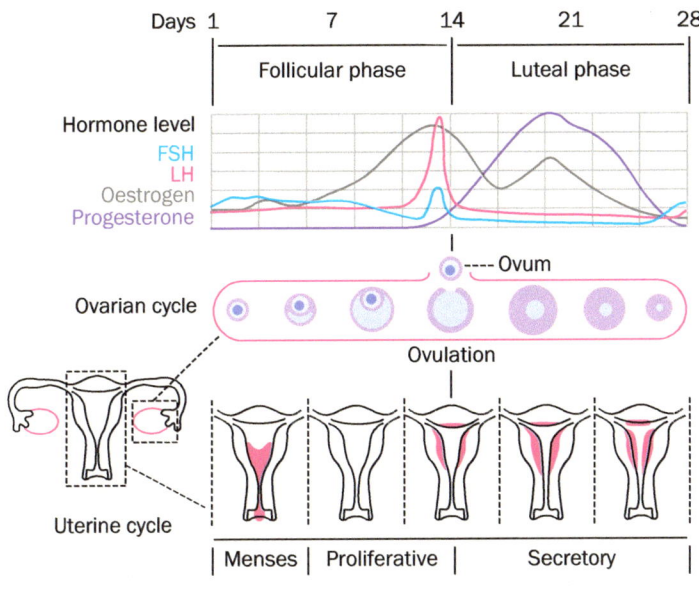

Figure 2.3 Stages of the menstrual cycle.

gestational calculator wheel if one is handy. It is important that this is seen as a guideline and not a definitive date as a number of factors can significantly influence the length of a pregnancy, including ethnicity, height, variations in the menstrual cycle, the timing of ovulation, parity and maternal weight (Wightman Lawson, 2021).

Contraception and fertility

Understanding the menstrual cycle is also important in order to discuss the most likely time for conception to take place and how contraceptive methods work. When patients are considering female sterilisation, it may be useful to share a diagram, such as Figure 2.2, to explain the occlusion of fallopian tubes.

Vaginal discharge

Understanding the physiology of normal vaginal discharge is an important starting point for identifying whether vaginal discharge needs treatment.

Glands inside the vagina and cervix produce small amounts of fluid known as vaginal secretions. The purpose of these secretions is to cleanse old cells that line the vagina to keep the vagina healthy. Some women have vaginal discharge every day, others less frequently, and it is important to know that vaginal discharge changes over the course of the menstrual cycle.

It is normal for women of reproductive age to have some degree of vaginal discharge. For women not on hormonal contraception, prior to ovulation, oestrogen levels increase, altering cervical mucus from thick and sticky (non-fertile and hostile to sperm) to clear, wet and slippery (fertile). When, after ovulation, progesterone levels begin to rise again and oestrogen levels fall, the vaginal discharge will become non-fertile again.

The vagina is colonised with commensal bacteria. Rising oestrogen levels at puberty lead to colonisation with lactobacilli which produce lactic acid. This means that the vaginal environment is acidic, with a pH of around 4.5. Some commensal organisms can cause a change in discharge if they 'overgrow'. This can lead to issues such as thrush (GP Notebook, 2021).

 For more information on changes in vaginal discharge see Table 7.1 on p. 86 in Chapter 7: Sexually Transmitted Infections.

■ The Male Reproductive System

The male reproductive system includes the penis and two testes. This, as well as some surrounding anatomy, is depicted in Figure 2.4.

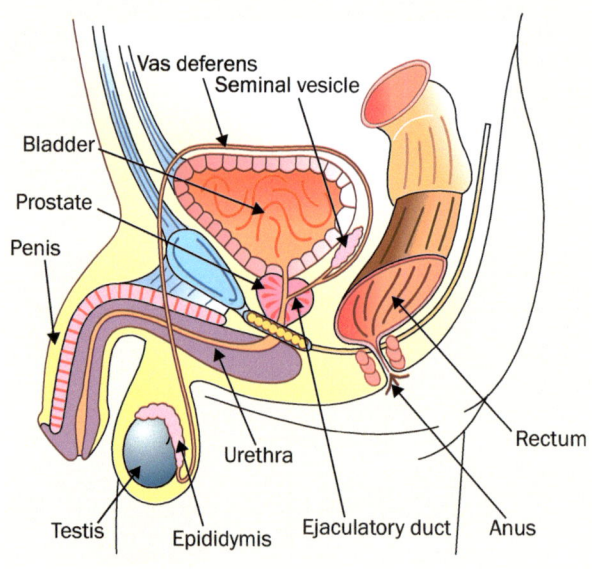

Figure 2.4 Male reproductive system.

CHAPTER 2 • Anatomy and Physiology – A Recap

Male fertility

A basic understanding of the male reproductive system, particularly sperm production and storage, is important when discussing male fertility and advice around vasectomy. It may be helpful to explain to patients the processes associated with sperm production and storage. Sperm are manufactured in the testes and stored both there and in the epididymis. They travel up the vas deferens, passing the seminal vesicles and the prostate gland. If the vas deferens is severed during vasectomy, the ejaculate is still formed by the seminal vesicles and the prostate gland. After vasectomy, the sperm are unable to get into the semen but the testes still make sperm; these are absorbed by the body without any harmful effects including detrimental changes to sexual response, arousal, orgasm or ejaculation. Patients may need reassurance that vasectomy will not decrease sex drive since the procedure does not affect the production of testosterone or the ability to get an erection or ejaculate.

■ External Genitalia: Documenting Anatomical Sites

There are a range of conditions including lesions, rashes, spots and blisters affecting external genitalia that are commonly referred to as 'spots, bumps and lumps'. Often these are variations of normal and all that will be needed is reassurance. HCPs need to be confident about describing the anatomical positioning of these when documenting, especially when referring on to other practitioners and in conversations with patients and colleagues.

Figures 2.5 and 2.6 provide a useful guide to naming the anatomy of external genitalia.

Increasingly with digital documentation, HCPs have access to templates or diagrams that can be used to identify the position of the area of concern. In the absence of these, many practitioners will draw a simple diagram in the patient's notes or on a piece of paper to enhance communication with other practitioners and/or explanations with the patient.

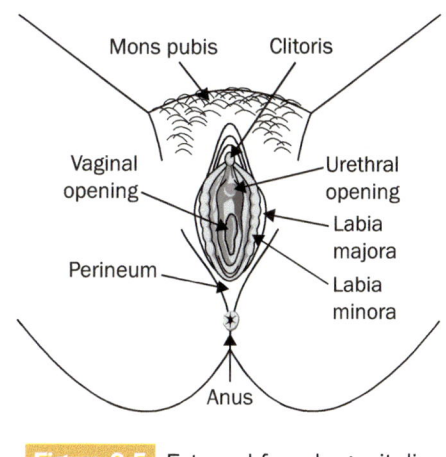

Figure 2.5 External female genitalia.

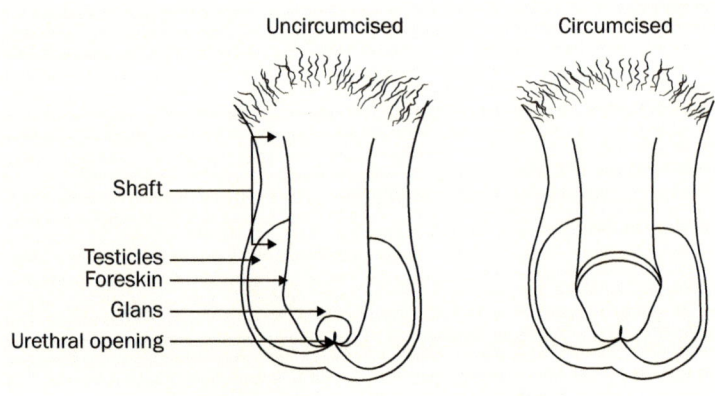

Figure 2.6 External male genitalia.

Concerns about appearance of external genitalia

It is common for patients to express concerns about the appearance of their genitalia. It is important that HCPs are able to reassure people about the range of normal variation in the appearance of external genitalia for both women and men.

> Here are some useful resources to share with colleagues and patients.
> - *What is a Vulva Anyway?* (BritSPAG, 2019). This booklet is designed to help readers understand their vulva and how puberty can change it. It explores worries that patients (particularly young patients) may have regarding their anatomy and highlights the fact that everyone is different.
> - *The Great Wall of Vulva*. Artist Jamie McCartney (2022) created The Great Wall of Vulva to demonstrate vulva diversity.
> - *Men's Health* (NHS, 2023). Includes common health questions such as: 'Is it normal to have a curved penis?' and 'What should my testicles look and feel like?'.
> - *Sexual Wellbeing for All* (2023).

> For more information on communication skills to aid effective consultations, including responding to concerns around sexual difficulties, see Chapter 1: Communication (pp. 1–12).

CHAPTER 3

Contraception

■ Introduction

Building the knowledge, skills, resilience and ambitions of young people, as well as providing easy access to welcoming services, helps them to delay sex until they are ready to enjoy healthy, consensual relationships and to use contraception effectively (PHE, 2018). Helping women to choose the method of contraception that suits them will help to reduce unplanned pregnancies (NICE, 2022a). To prevent unintended pregnancies, contraception needs to be used up until the menopause.

This chapter will follow the current Faculty of Sexual and Reproductive Healthcare UK Medical Eligibility Criteria (FSRH, 2016), the British Association for Sexual Health and HIV guidance (BASHH, 2021) and relevant National Institute for Health and Care Excellence (NICE) guidance throughout. Current local guidelines should also be followed.

■ Faculty of Sexual and Reproductive Healthcare UK Medical Eligibility Criteria

When offering contraception, it is important to refer to the FSRH UK Medical Eligibility Criteria for Contraceptive Use (UKMEC), which offers guidance on who can use contraceptive methods safely. These are evidence-based recommendations that allow for consideration of the possible methods that can be used safely by individuals based on medical conditions and personal characteristics (FSRH, 2016).

■ History Taking and Consultation

Along with the UKMEC and determining the safest contraceptive method for the patient to use, you must also discuss all the available contraceptive options with the patient and consider what might best fit their lifestyle. For example, it may not be ideal for a cabin crew worker to start the combined oral contraceptive pill (COCP), as working in shifts across different time zones will make it difficult to know when to take their next pill. In this case, a long-acting reversible contraceptive (LARC) would be more suitable. On the other hand, the patient may want to get pregnant within the next year and therefore a LARC method, such as an intrauterine contraceptive (IUC), may not be suitable for them. To allow patients to take their time when considering their choice, it may be useful to provide written information. You can point them in the direction of the Sexwise website where this information is freely available.

What to ask when taking a history
Contraception and sexual history
- Is the patient already on a method of contraception?
- Has there been any contraception failure, such as missed pills or a damaged condom, that could increase pregnancy risk? If so, discuss and offer emergency contraception (EC).
- Establish the reason for the patient wanting to start or switch contraception.
  - Is there a new sexual partner?
  - Is it due to menstrual-related issues?
  - Are there any side-effects with the current contraception, for example mood changes?
- If this is a new partner, offer STI screening. If appropriate (if the patient is under the age of 18), ask what age their partner is.
- Ask if the sex is consensual, free from coercion and that the patient is happy in their sexual relationship (you should consult with the patient alone to ask this).
- If the patient is asking for a repeat prescription of a pill, check that they are remembering to take the pill. It can be helpful to ask the patient in an open way, such as 'How many pills have you missed this month?'. Discuss ways of remembering such as setting an alarm or putting the pill pack by their toothbrush.
- Does the patient have a preference of which contraceptive method they would like to use? Patients often read online about the different methods before contacting you, so this can be a useful starting point. A discussion of the advantages and disadvantages of each method in relation to the patient's personal circumstances should take place.
- Ask questions in relation to the specific contraceptive method and the UKMEC to ensure the method the patient wishes to start is safe for them to have.
- If the patient is over the age of 25, it is important that you check whether their smear is up to date during the consultation.
- When starting a new method, always give the individual an NHS patient information leaflet (PIL) or refer to the appropriate website regarding their contraceptive method. This will include details on what to do if there is a missed pill or adverse effects and can serve as a good reminder for patients (NHS, 2019).

CHAPTER 3 • Contraception

Medical history
- Does the patient have any medical conditions?
- Are they taking any regular medicines?
- Do they have any drug allergies?

Menstrual history
- Ask about the patient's LMP, their cycle length, whether there is a pattern, heavy and/or painful periods or anything else of note.

Obstetric history
- Any previous pregnancies? If so, the outcome of these, for example miscarriage, abortion, live birth (include year/years).
- Were the births vaginal deliveries or caesarean section?
- Does the patient have any children? How old are they?

Drug history
- Ask about any current prescription, non-prescription or recreational drugs.

Family history
- Any relevant family history, in particular ischaemic heart disease, venous thromboembolism (VTE), breast cancer and ovarian cancer.

Social history
- Alcohol and smoking or vaping.
- Occupation.

Ensure you are aware of local policies on how to escalate encounters where patients disclose problems with sexual relationships, such as non-consensual sex or sexual violence.

■ Examination

Depending on each individual's situation and which contraceptive method they are opting for, you may need to take their blood pressure, a body mass index (BMI) (record height and weight) and an up-to-date pregnancy test. At least a routine annual review is recommended by the FSRH, but this can be reduced to six monthly if the clinician is concerned (for example, due to age, safeguarding or weight).

Further reading regarding ensuring the method of contraception is safe can be found within the UKMEC guidelines (FSRH, 2016).

Types of Contraception

There is no evidence of weight gain for any of the contraceptive methods apart from the Depo-Provera® injection as it can increase appetite. Hormonal contraception may be associated with mood changes but there is no evidence that hormonal contraceptives cause depression.

Progestogen-only pill

The progestogen-only pill (POP) can also be referred to as the 'mini pill', but this is a colloquial term which can be misleading and therefore it is preferred that HCPs do not use it.

Effectiveness
The POP is 99% effective if taken correctly, but with typical use it is around 91% effective.

How it works
It is a progestogen-only method of contraception and works primarily by thickening cervical mucus and thinning the lining of the uterus (FPA, 2020). In addition, the desogestrel POP inhibits ovulation.

Advantages
The POP is well suited for women who want to take a pill as a method but are contraindicated or prefer not to take oestrogen.

The POP has fewer risks than the COCP for certain conditions such as blood clots and breast cancer. For example, women are still able to take the POP if they are overweight, smoke or suffer with migraines.

Disadvantages
A disadvantage of the POP is that it commonly causes irregular bleeding, particularly in the first 3–6 months, and may continue to cause bleeding issues after this time (although often bleeding stops altogether). Additionally, if the patient has diarrhoea and vomiting, then the POP may not be fully effective. Often, women report side-effects of acne and breast pain, so this particular method may not be suitable for women who already suffer with spots.

How to use and effect on fertility
The POP can be taken up until the age of 55 (FSRH, 2019a). It is taken continuously once a day, without a break for a withdrawal bleed. There are

CHAPTER 3 · Contraception

two different types of POP; the most commonly used is desogestrel, which must be taken within 12 hours of the same time each day. There is also the 'traditional' POP, such as norethisterone, which should be taken within three hours of the same time each day. There are 28 pills in a POP pack (Figure 3.1). When a patient finishes a pack, they simply start the next pack. If the patient starts the POP on day 1–5 of their menstrual cycle, it will work straight away and they will be protected against pregnancy. If they start the POP on any other day of their cycle, they will not be protected from pregnancy straight away and will need to avoid sexual intercourse or use additional barrier methods of contraception until they have taken the pill for two days (48 hours).

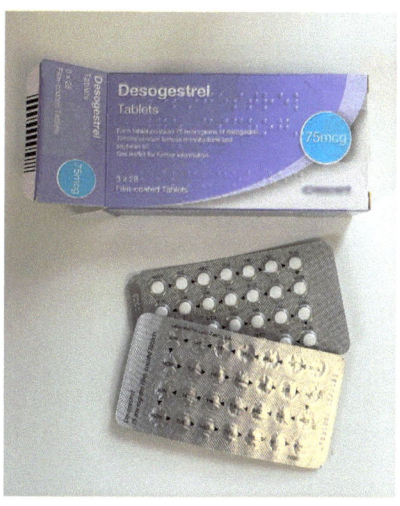

Figure 3.1 POP.

If the patient has just had a baby, they can start the POP on day 21 after the birth and they will be protected against pregnancy straight away. If they start the POP more than 21 days after giving birth, they will need to use additional barrier methods of contraception until they have taken the pill for two days (NHS, 2021a).

 Specific advice is required for patients who miss taking their pill, which is available from the NHS (2021a).

Long-acting reversible contraception

In 2005, NICE published its guideline on LARC, with an aim to increase their use because their effectiveness does not depend on the woman remembering to take or use them. In addition, the NICE guideline and quality standard on contraception recommend that women asking for contraception are given information about, and offered a choice of, all methods of contraception including LARC (NHS, 2018b). Since this publication, user-dependent contraceptives, such as the oral contraceptive pill, have gradually decreased over time, from 77% in 2007 to 59% in 2018. During the same time, use of LARC methods has increased from 23% to 41% (NICE, 2022a).

Contraceptive injection

Women now have the option of both Depo-Provera (Figure 3.2) and Sayana® Press. Sayana Press is a self-administered subcutaneous injection that

23

patients are able to give themselves at home, once they have been shown how to do it by a clinician. This suits many women due to the convenience of administering in your own home in your own time, but others do not like the idea of self-injecting and prefer to opt for Depo-Provera. Discuss both options with your patient, so that they can make an informed choice.

Effectiveness

With careful use, the contraceptive injection is over 99% effective, but typical use results in around 94% effectiveness, as sometimes injections are administered late (FPA, 2020).

How it works

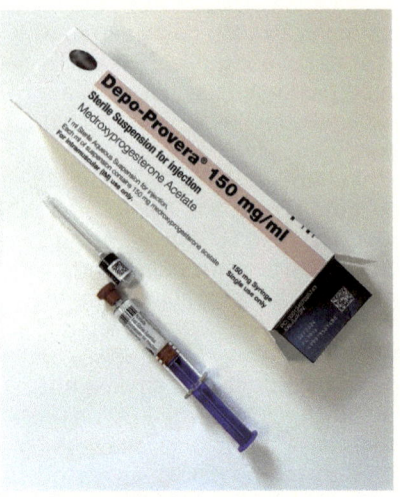

Figure 3.2 Depo-Provera.

The contraceptive injection is a progestogen-only contraceptive, which works by releasing progestogen to stop ovulation, thickening cervical mucus to prevent sperm reaching an egg and thinning the lining of the uterus to prevent a fertilised egg implanting.

Advantages

It lasts for 13 weeks and can be very effective at reducing heavy periods (often bleeding completely stops). There is also no requirement for the patient to remember to take a pill daily.

Disadvantages

Disadvantages of the contraceptive injection can include unpredictable and irregular bleeding and weight gain. Additionally, it is vital to inform your patient that periods and fertility can take a year to return after stopping the injection, which is important if they want to conceive soon. Moreover, as it is injected into the bloodstream, it cannot be removed, so any side-effects may continue until it is out of the patient's system. Women need to receive the injection every 13 weeks for it to be fully effective.

Several studies have shown that bone density decreases by a small amount in women who use this contraceptive method (Dennerstein et al., 2018). Therefore, it is essential that women are asked about any family history of osteoporosis, any personal history of fractures or anorexia nervosa and whether they smoke. If the answer is 'yes' it would be worth discussing an alternative option.

CHAPTER 3 · Contraception

How to use and effect on fertility
It can be given at any time during the cycle as long as the woman is not pregnant or at risk of pregnancy. If the injection is given in the first five days of a cycle, the patient will be protected against pregnancy straight away. If it is given at any other time, it is vital to inform the patient to use additional contraception, such as condoms, for seven days afterwards or abstain from sexual intercourse.

Contraceptive implant
Effectiveness
The implant is highly effective at preventing pregnancy, with over 99% efficacy (FPA, 2020).

How it works
It involves a small flexible rod (Figure 3.3) that is put under the skin of the upper arm. This releases the progestogen hormone, which stops ovulation, thickens cervical mucus to prevent sperm from reaching an egg and thins the lining of the uterus, to prevent an egg implanting.

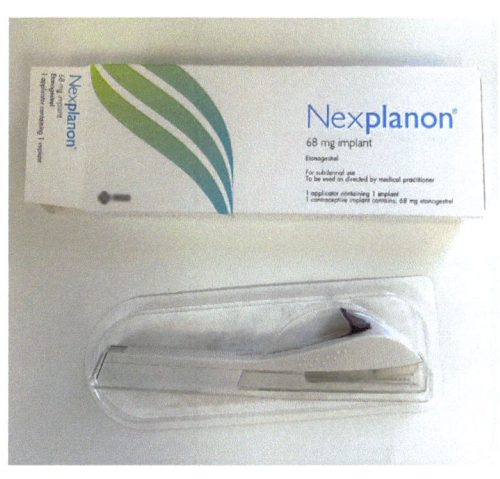

Figure 3.3 The implant.

Advantages
Advantages of the implant include not needing to remember a pill/patch, and once it is removed, fertility returns to normal instantly. According to the UKMEC, it is viewed as one of the safest contraceptives. Most primary care providers fit contraceptive implants.

Disadvantages
Disadvantages of the implant include irregular and unpredictable bleeding patterns and the requirement of a small procedure to fit and remove it (inserted using a local anaesthetic, no stitches required). The patient may be left with a small scar and the implant can cause or worsen acne in some women (Ramdhan et al., 2018). The patient should be advised that they should be able to feel the implant, but not see it.

How to use and effect on fertility
Once it is fitted, it works for three years, although it can be removed sooner if a patient is getting unwanted side-effects or wishes to conceive. It can be

25

fitted at any point during the menstrual cycle as long as the patient is not pregnant. If it is fitted during the first five days of the menstrual cycle then it is effective immediately. If fitted on any other day of the menstrual cycle, advise the patient to abstain from sexual intercourse or use another form of contraception (condoms) for seven days.

Intrauterine contraception

The IUC is highly effective and long acting, making it a very cost-effective option (FPA, 2020). There are two main types: levonorgestrel intrauterine system (LNG-IUS) (Figure 3.4) and copper intrauterine device (Cu-IUD).

The LNG-IUS

Mirena® is the leading brand and is the only intrauterine system (IUS) licensed to be used as the progestogen component of hormone replacement therapy (HRT). Many primary care providers have trained practitioners who can fit IUSs within the practice, or it may be commissioned outside primary care within local sexual health clinics.

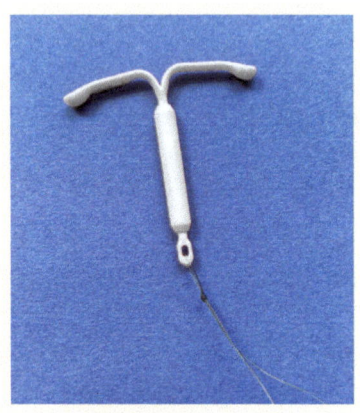

Figure 3.4 LNG-IUS.

Effectiveness
The LNG-IUS is over 99% effective and once it is fitted, it works as a contraceptive for 3–8 years depending on the type (Mirena: 8 years) (FSRH, 2024). If the LNG-IUS is fitted under the age of 45, it works as a contraceptive for up to 8 years. If it is inserted over 45 years, it can be used as a contraceptive until the age of 55. It is important to note that the LNG-IUS can only be used for five years as endometrial protection as part of HRT (FSRH, 2023a).

How it works
The LNG-IUS is a small, flexible T-shaped plastic device which is inserted into the uterus where it releases progestogen. It works by thinning the lining of the uterus to stop a fertilised egg implanting and thickens the cervical mucus so that it is difficult for sperm to reach the egg. In some women it also supresses ovarian function.

Advantages
The effect the LNG-IUS has on bleeding varies from woman to woman; bleeding usually becomes lighter and less painful, and it may completely stop. However, many women do suffer with unpredictable and irregular bleeding in the first six months.

CHAPTER 3 • Contraception

Disadvantages
Insertion can be uncomfortable or painful (FPA, 2020). Numerous studies and systematic reviews have sought effective strategies to reduce pain associated with IUC insertion, but there is no clear superior analgesic option. Ketoprofen or naproxen taken an hour before the procedure could be beneficial for insertion and post-insertion pain. There is no evidence for routine prophylactic use of ibuprofen, although non-steroidal anti-inflammatory drugs (NSAIDs) are beneficial for treating established pain after insertion (FSRH, 2021).

How to use and effect on fertility
The LNG-IUS can be fitted any time in the menstrual cycle as long as the patient is not pregnant or at recent risk of pregnancy. If it is fitted in the first seven days of a cycle, the patient will be protected against pregnancy straight away. If it is fitted at any other time, it is vital to inform the patient to use additional contraception, such as condoms, for seven days afterwards, or to abstain from sexual intercourse (FSRH, 2016). When the LNG-IUS is removed, the patient's fertility will return to normal instantly.

Copper IUD
Effectiveness
The Cu-IUD (Figure 3.5) is over 99% effective and once it is fitted, it works as a contraceptive for 5–10 years depending on the type (usually 10 years). It is the gold standard of EC and can be fitted up to five days from the earliest predicted ovulation.

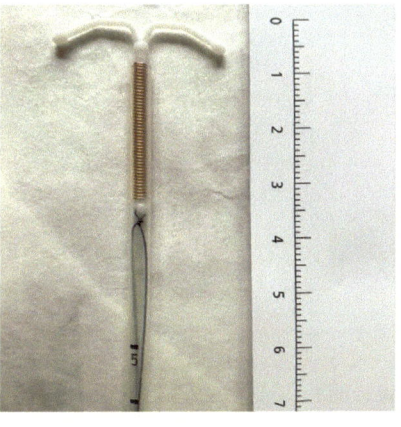

Figure 3.5 Cu-IUD.

 For further information see Chapter 4: Emergency Contraception (pp. 41–53)

How it works
A small, flexible, plastic and copper device is inserted into the uterus. The copper impairs the viability of sperm and eggs and changes cervical mucus to stop sperm from being able to reach the egg.

Advantages
An obvious advantage of the Cu-IUD for many women is that it does not use any hormones.

Disadvantages

A disadvantage is that it can make periods heavier and more painful (the patient will still have regular monthly bleeds), making it an unsuitable method if the patient already suffers with dysmenorrhoea and menorrhagia.

How to use and effect on fertility

It starts working as soon as it has been inserted (no need to use extra precautions for seven days afterwards) and the patient's fertility will return to normal as soon as the Cu-IUD is removed.

Both IUC methods have a very small chance of an infection occurring within the first 20 days after insertion (FPA, 2020). IUC users should also be informed about symptoms of ectopic pregnancy. The possibility of ectopic pregnancy should be considered in women with an IUC method who present with abdominal pain, especially in connection with missed periods or if an amenorrhoeic woman starts bleeding. If a pregnancy test is positive, an ultrasound scan (USS) is urgently required to locate the pregnancy. There is also a very small risk of perforating the womb, which occurs in 1 in 1000 insertions (Rowlands et al., 2016).

Combined methods of contraception

Combined oral contraceptive pill

There are several different brands of COCP available (Figure 3.6), each with different doses of oestrogen/type of progestogen. It can be trial and error finding out which COCP works best for each woman in relation to their mood/skin and bleeding patterns. The brands available are constantly changing. If you are a prescriber, you should follow both the FSRH and local guidance.

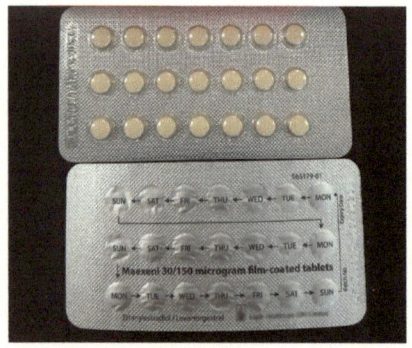

Figure 3.6 COCP.

Effectiveness
The COCP is 99% effective if used correctly, but with typical use it is around 91% effective (FPA, 2020).

The antibiotics rifampicin and rifabutin (which can be used to treat tuberculosis and meningitis) can reduce the effectiveness of the COCP. Other antibiotics do not have this effect. The COCP can also interact with enzyme inducers. These speed up the breakdown of hormones by the liver, reducing the effectiveness of the pill. Examples include carbamazepine, rifampicin, phenytoin and St John's wort (Simmons et al., 2018).

How it works
It is a combined method and therefore includes two hormones (oestrogen and progestogen). It works by stopping ovulation, thickening cervical mucus to prevent sperm reaching an egg and thinning the lining of the uterus to prevent an egg implanting.

Advantages
Use of the COCP may be associated with non-contraceptive health benefits, particularly reducing heavy bleeding, lessening painful periods and improving acne. Additionally, use of the COCP is associated with a significant reduction in the risk of endometrial and ovarian cancer (FPA, 2020). A clear advantage of the COCP is that a woman can have more control over her monthly bleeds.

Disadvantages
Missing pills, vomiting or severe diarrhoea can make the COCP less effective.

Due to the COCP being a combined method of contraception, it is vital to ask the patient questions in relation to the UKMEC. Combined methods of contraception can be associated with blood clots and breast cancer (still a relatively low risk) and the patient should be made aware of these risks (FSRH, 2023b).

Combined hormonal contraception (CHC) is associated with a very small increased risk of myocardial infarction and ischaemic stroke that appears to be greater with higher doses of oestrogen. Due to these risks, the COCP is not suitable for women who:

- smoke and are over the age of 35
- are over the age of 50
- have (or have ever experienced) migraine with aura
- are obese (BMI over 35)
- have hypertension

- have a history of VTE or a first-degree relative with a history of VTE under the age of 45
- have a history of breast cancer.

 Refer to the UKMEC (FSRH, 2016) for a full list of personal characteristics and medical conditions.

How to use and effect on fertility

Traditionally, women on the COCP take a seven-day break at the end of each 21-pill packet. During this monthly break from pill taking, there is usually a bleed, and some women have symptoms such as menstrual cramps, headache and mood change. However, a new NICE-accredited clinical guideline from the FSRH highlights that there is no health benefit from having this hormone-free interval (FSRH, 2023b). Women can avoid monthly bleeding and any associated symptoms by running pill packets together so that they take fewer, or no, breaks. If a hormone-free interval is taken, shortening it to four days could potentially reduce the risk of pregnancy if pills are missed (FSRH, 2023b). However, by not having the seven-day break, women may report 'spotting' or irregular and unpredictable bleeding. Women should be given information about both standard and tailored regimens to broaden contraceptive choice. However, they should be advised that the use of tailored regimens is outside the manufacturer's licence but is supported by the FSRH. The different ways of taking the COCP are summarised in Table 3.1.

Table 3.1 Standard and tailored regimens for CHC.*

Regimen	CHC length of use	Hormone-free interval
Standard	21 days	7 days
Shortened	21 days	4 days
Extended (*tricycling)	9 weeks* or 6 weeks consecutive	4 or 7 days
Flexible	Continuous ≥21 days until breakthrough bleeding occurs for 3–4 days	4–7 days
Continuous	Continuous	None

Source: FSRH (2023b).
*Note: this includes pills, patches and the contraceptive ring.

 More information about the COCP can be found at Sexwise (2021).

The COCP needs to be taken at around the same time every day. If the patient starts their combined pill on the first day of their period, up to and including the fifth day of their period, they will be protected from pregnancy straight away and will not need additional contraception. However, if the pill is commenced after this date, then they will not be protected from pregnancy straight away and will need to abstain from sexual intercourse or use additional barrier methods of contraception until they have taken the pill for seven days.

If the patient vomits within three hours of taking the COCP, it may not have been fully absorbed, and the patient should be advised to take another pill straight away and the next pill at their usual time. If they continue to vomit, they should use another form of contraception until they have taken the pill again for seven days without vomiting/severe diarrhoea.

If the patient has just had a baby, they are not breastfeeding and do not have any other risk factors, they can most likely start the pill on day 21 after the birth. They will be protected against pregnancy straight away. If they start the COCP later than 21 days after giving birth, they will need additional contraception for the next seven days. If the woman is breastfeeding, it is not advised to take the COCP until six weeks after the birth (FSRH, 2016). Fertility returns to normal once the COCP is stopped.

 Specific advice is required for patients who miss taking their COCP, which is available from the NHS (2019).

Combined transdermal patch
Effectiveness
The combined transdermal patch is 99% effective if used correctly, but with typical use it is around 91% effective (FPA, 2020).

How it works
It is a small patch, approximately 5 × 5 cm (Figure 3.7), that adheres to the skin and releases both oestrogen and progestogen, which stops ovulation, thickens cervical mucus to prevent sperm reaching an egg and thins the lining of the uterus to prevent an egg implanting.

Advantages
Advantages of the patch include not needing to remember a pill every day, but still offering the benefits of a combined hormonal method. Additionally, it is not affected if the patient has diarrhoea or vomiting, and the patient can determine their monthly bleeds by running patches together. It often makes periods less painful and lighter.

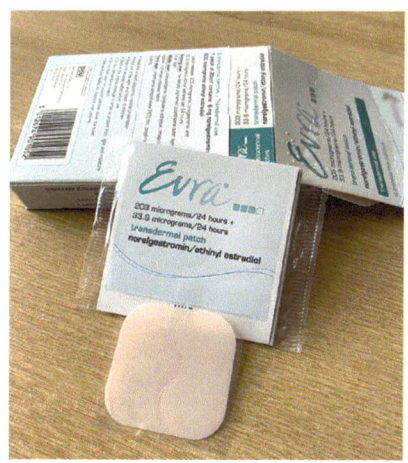

Figure 3.7 Combined transdermal patch.

Disadvantages

A disadvantage of the patch is that it can be visible, making it less discreet. Limited evidence suggests a possible reduction in patch effectiveness in women ≥90 kg, and therefore alternatives should be used if the patient is over 90 kg (FSRH, 2019b).

 Due to the contraceptive patch being a combined method of contraception, it is vital to ask the patient questions in relation to the UKMEC.

How to use and effect on fertility

Table 3.1 also applies for the different ways of using the contraceptive patch. However, the traditional way of taking the patch involves applying the first patch and wearing it for seven days. On day eight, the patient will need to change the patch to a new one. They will need to change it like this every week for three weeks, and then have a patch-free week. During the patch-free week, they will get a withdrawal bleed, although this may not always happen. After seven patch-free days, the patient should apply a new patch and start the four-week cycle again.

If the patient starts using the patch on the first day of their period, and up to and including the fifth day of their period, they will be protected from pregnancy straight away. If they start using it on any other day, they need to use an additional form of contraception for the first seven days, or abstain from sexual intercourse (NHS, 2021b). The patch can be worn in the bath, when swimming and while playing sports and can be applied to most areas of the body apart from the breasts.

 Specific advice is required for patients who forget to take their patch off or put a new one on after the patch-free week, which is available from the NHS (2021b).

Combined vaginal ring

Effectiveness

The combined vaginal ring is 99% effective if always used according to instructions, but with typical use it is 91% effective (FPA, 2020).

How it works

It involves the woman inserting a small, flexible plastic ring into the vagina, where it releases both oestrogen and progestogen (the vaginal ring is a combined hormonal method of contraception) (Figure 3.8). It works by stopping ovulation, thickening the cervical mucus to stop sperm reaching the egg and thinning the lining of the uterus to stop an egg implanting.

CHAPTER 3 • Contraception

 Due to the vaginal ring being a combined hormonal method of contraception, it is vital to ask the patient questions in relation to the UKMEC.

Advantages
The patient can continue to have sex as usual when the ring is in place; a partner may feel it, but this is not harmful. Unlike the pill, the ring still works even if the patient has vomiting and diarrhoea. For most women, the ring lightens bleeding and makes periods less painful. For women who suffer with acne, the vaginal ring may improve their skin.

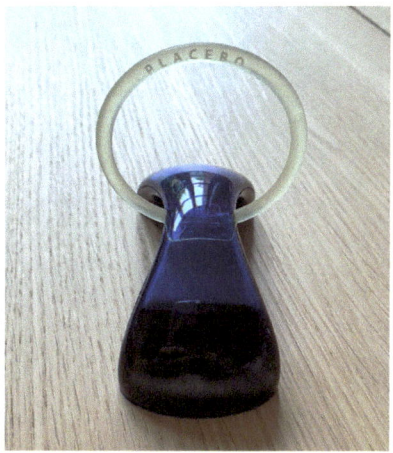

Figure 3.8 Combined vaginal ring.

Disadvantages
Occasionally, the ring can come out on its own, but it can be rinsed with warm water and reinserted within three hours without the need to use additional contraception.

How to use and effect on fertility
One ring provides contraception for a month. The patient can start using the vaginal ring at any time during their menstrual cycle as long as they are not pregnant. See the COCP section for different ways of using the contraceptive vaginal ring (Table 3.1). Traditionally, the patient needs to leave the ring in for 21 days, then remove it and have a seven-day ring-free break. They are protected against pregnancy during the ring-free break. A new ring is then inserted for another 21 days. The patient will be protected against pregnancy straight away if the ring is inserted on the first day of their period (information on how to insert the ring is given in Box 3.1). If the patient starts using the ring at any other time in their menstrual cycle, they will need to use additional contraception for the first seven days of using it, or abstain from sexual intercourse.

Box 3.1 How to insert a vaginal ring

To insert the ring, the patient will need to clean their hands, squeeze the ring between their thumb and finger and gently insert the tip into the vagina, gently pushing the ring up until it feels comfortable. To remove the ring, the patient will need to clean their hands, put a finger into their vagina and hook it around the edge of the ring, gently pulling the ring out. It can then be put it in the special bag provided and disposed of in the bin, advising not to flush it down the toilet. Removing the ring should be painless (NHS, 2021c).

Specific advice for patients who forget to take the ring out or forget to insert a new ring is available from the NHS (2021c).

Barrier methods
Condoms
It is important to offer condoms to patients when they come to see you for any kind of sexual health or contraceptive issue (particularly if they are under the age of 25). Female (internal) condoms are also available, though these are not as widely available as male (external) condoms. They are made from soft, thin synthetic latex or polyurethane. Both are worn to prevent semen getting to the womb and are 95% effective (NHS, 2020a, 2021d).

 Condom distribution schemes are often commissioned, so ensure your practice knows how to access 'free' stock.

Effectiveness
If used correctly and consistently, condoms can be 98% effective although with typical use, around 18 in 100 women will become pregnant every year when using condoms as the only form of contraception (FPA, 2020).

Advantages
The methods of contraception previously discussed do not offer protection from STIs. However, as a barrier method, condoms help protect both partners from some STIs, including HIV. Non-hormonal contraception is becoming increasingly popular as an option for couples. Condoms are available in a range of sizes and do not come with any serious side-effects (apart from latex allergy).

Disadvantages
The biggest issue with condoms is that they can sometimes split or slip off, particularly if the incorrect size is used. This can result in a woman requiring EC.

 If possible, avoid using spermicidal lubricated condoms because they commonly contain a chemical called nonoxinol-9, which may increase the risk of HIV and other infections (FPA, 2020).

How to use
Condoms are made from very thin latex (rubber), polyurethane (plastic) or polyisoprene and simply cover an erect penis to prevent sperm from entering the vagina.

Diaphragms
Diaphragms are non-hormonal barrier methods of contraception that protect women against pregnancy by preventing sperm reaching the cervix. The Caya®

is the most common and comes in one single size (it will accommodate 80% of women).

Effectiveness
When used correctly with spermicide, a diaphragm, or cap, is 92–96% effective at preventing pregnancy.

Advantages
A diaphragm only needs to be used when about to engage in sexual intercourse. There are no associated health risks.

Disadvantages
It is possible to develop a urinary tract infection (UTI) when using a diaphragm; switching to a smaller size may help. Latex and spermicide can cause irritation for either sexual partner. It can also take practice to learn how to use a diaphragm correctly.

How to use
Insert a diaphragm with spermicide before having sex. Extra spermicide should be added if the diaphragm has been in place for more than three hours. The diaphragm or cap needs to be left in place for at least six hours after sexual intercourse.

Condoms should be considered in addition to enhance protection against STIs.

Vasectomy

A vasectomy is more than 99% effective. It is a surgical procedure to seal the tubes that carry sperm, permanently preventing pregnancy. Sperm is prevented from entering the semen so when ejaculation occurs, the semen has no sperm to fertilise an egg. It is considered permanent and is very difficult to reverse, so it is important to ensure it is the right choice for your patient.

The patient will need to use contraception for at least 8–12 weeks after the operation, because sperm will still be in the tubes leading to the penis.

Female sterilisation

Female sterilisation is an operation to permanently prevent pregnancy. The fallopian tubes are blocked or sealed to prevent the eggs reaching the sperm and becoming fertilised. Eggs will still be released from the ovaries as normal, but they will be absorbed naturally into the woman's body. It is very difficult to reverse and therefore counselling is recommended to ensure the right choice for the patient.

Sexual Health and Contraception

 Female sterilisation does not affect hormone levels and the patient will still have periods.

 It is recommended that both patient and partner agree with vasectomy or female sterilisation, but it is not a legal requirement to have partner permission.

■ Contraceptive Choices and Sexual Health for Transgender and Non-Binary People

The FSRH has specific guidance on contraception for trans people. In general, combined hormonal methods are not suitable for trans men and non-binary people who take testosterone, but progestogen-only methods, the IUS and EC can all be used.

It should be noted that trans people may or may not elect to seek medical help and that, if sought, this medical help is highly individualised. Individuals' goals from hormone use and surgery vary and therefore so will the appropriateness and acceptability of different methods of contraception. Sensitive communication is key, with a clear attempt to avoid any stigmatising language (FSRH, 2017).

 For more on this see pp. 11–12 in Chapter 1: Communication.

The FSRH (2017) gives the following guidelines for transgender and non-binary people and contraception.

- There is no restriction on the use of any method of contraception for people assigned female at birth on account of their current gender identity. People who were assigned female at birth should be given information about all methods of contraception for which they are medically eligible and helped to decide which would suit their needs.
- For trans men and non-binary (assigned female) people who have not undergone hysterectomy or bilateral oophorectomy having vaginal sex and not wishing to conceive, contraception is recommended.
- Testosterone treatment does not provide adequate contraceptive protection.
- Gonadotrophin-releasing hormone (GnRH) analogues cannot be relied on for contraceptive protection. Pregnancy is an absolute contraindication to testosterone therapy.
- If pregnancy does occur, testosterone treatment used in current regimens can be associated with teratogenicity.
- Cu-IUDs are safe to use and do not interfere with hormone regimens.
- Progestogen-only contraceptive methods are not thought to interfere with hormone regimens.

CHAPTER 3 • Contraception

- Use of CHCs by those undergoing testosterone treatment is not recommended as the oestrogen component of CHCs will counteract the masculinising effects of testosterone.
- Trans women and non-binary (assigned male) people who have not undergone orchidectomy or vasectomy should ensure that effective contraception is used if they are having vaginal sex and their partner does not wish to conceive.
- A trans woman or non-binary person who is receiving oestradiol therapy should be aware that although oestradiol treatment results in impaired spermatogenesis, it does not provide adequate contraceptive protection if they are having vaginal sex.
- A trans woman or non-binary person who is receiving hormonal therapy should be aware that these treatments cannot be relied on for contraceptive protection to reduce or block sperm production.

Health Promotion

Contraception after childbirth

Fertility may return quickly, so it is important for post-partum women to be offered contraception at the earliest point possible to reduce the risk of unintended pregnancies. It is possible to fall pregnant after day 21 post-partum. Moreover, providing advice about contraception after childbirth helps avoid the risk of complications associated with an interpregnancy interval of less than 12 months (NICE, 2016).

 Contraception After Pregnancy (FSRH, 2020a).

Breastfeeding

Breastfeeding can be 98% effective at preventing pregnancy up to six months after giving birth if the woman is exclusively breastfeeding (day and night), their baby is up to six months old and they have not yet had a period (Tiwari et al., 2018). This is known as lactational amenorrhea (LAM). Women using LAM should be advised that the risk of pregnancy is increased if the frequency of breastfeeding decreases, when menstruation returns or at more than six months after childbirth (FSRH, 2020a).

Opportunities for health promotion

 Thirty percent of pregnant women under the age of 20 reported being a smoker at their first booking appointment, and 37% of women under 20 years are overweight or obese in early pregnancy (AYPH, 2021). Discussing contraceptives with patients can be an excellent opportunity for health promotion, particularly when initiating any combined method of contraception.

In 2017, rates of conceptions in the under-18 age group were at their lowest level since 1969, but the UK still has a relatively high rate of births among 15–19 year olds compared with other similar high-income countries (NICE, 2022a). Understanding the law relating to conversations with patients less than 18 years of age is important.

See Chapter 8: Safeguarding, for more information on the law relating to young people.

Contraceptive Choices for Young people (FSRH, 2010).

CASE STUDY

Presenting complaint
You are working in a primary care practice and a 20-year-old female patient presents to you asking to start the pill.

History

History of presenting complaint
- She tells you that she has never been on contraception before.
- She tells you that she has never been sexually active and that there is no chance of pregnancy.
- She is happy in her relationship and wants to begin having a sexual relationship with her new partner.
- Her partner is also 20 years old and has had five previous sexual partners.
- When asked why the contraceptive pill as a method, she says she is not aware of other options available to her.
- She has no family history of breast cancer or VTE.
- She does not suffer with migraines.
- She suffers with acne.
- She suffers with what she describes as 'quite heavy and painful' periods that can be irregular at times.

Past medical history
None.

Social/family/drug history
- She is currently at university studying agriculture and does not work any night shifts.
- She is a non-smoker.

CHAPTER 3 • Contraception

Examination
- She appears well and you do not have any safeguarding concerns.
- Her blood pressure is 122/76.
- Her BMI is 22.

Management plan
- You discuss the different options for contraception with her, including LARC and both options of the contraceptive pill, as well as the contraceptive patch. You have a shared discussion on the best method for her, taking into consideration the pros and cons of each method for her personal circumstances. She tells you that she would prefer to start the COCP. You make her aware of the low risk of blood clots and breast cancer, but also the benefits of the COCP for her personal circumstances. You deem that she can clearly understand and retain information and use that information to make an informed decision.
- She has a UKMEC score of 1 and there are no contraindications to commencing on the COCP.
- You inform her of the different ways in which she can take the COCP. She decides to tricycle her packs due to her heavy and painful periods. She is aware that she needs to take the pill at the same time every day.
- Her period is not due for around three weeks, so you advise her that she can 'quick start' her pill, as she is likely to be sexually active and at risk of pregnancy very soon. You make it very clear that the COCP will not be effective for seven days and that extra precautions (such as condoms or abstaining from sexual intercourse) must be taken to prevent pregnancy risk.
- You discuss 'missed pill rules' with her and ensure understanding.
- You provide her with either a written PIL or a link to a PIL.
- As it is within your scope of practice, you prescribe six months of the COCP initially and then ask her to book a review in advance of that date, to ensure she does not run out of pills.
- As her partner has been sexually active before, you discuss the importance of STI screening. She agrees and takes a chlamydia screening pack and instructions from you.
- Before she leaves, you ask her if she has any further questions, or anything she would like you to repeat.

CHAPTER 4

Emergency Contraception

■ Introduction

Requests for emergency contraception (EC) are a common presentation in primary care. It is vital to take a full sexual history when consulting with a woman asking for EC. Some patients may find the process of acquiring EC quite distressing and/or embarrassing. Therefore, it is important to build a good rapport, make the patient feel as comfortable as possible and explore their need for EC. EC is available from:

- primary care services
- pharmacies (for those over the age of 16)
- sexual health clinics
- NHS walk-in centres
- EDs (although it is inappropriate to suggest this as an alternative care pathway and not all EDs will offer EC).

■ Indications for Emergency Contraception

Emergency contraception should be offered if a woman has had unprotected sexual intercourse (UPSI) on any day of her natural menstrual cycle, or if she thinks her contraception may have failed and she does not wish to conceive (FSRH, 2020b). This is because pregnancy is theoretically possible after UPSI on most days of the cycle, although risk of pregnancy is highest after UPSI which takes place during the six days leading up to and including the day of ovulation.

It is important to note that EC should be offered to any woman who does not wish to conceive and has had UPSI from day 21 after childbirth (unless the criteria for LAM have been met).

 For more on LAM, go to p. 37 in Chapter 3: Contraception.

Sexual Health and Contraception

Emergency contraception should also be offered when UPSI has taken place from day five after abortion, miscarriage, ectopic pregnancy or uterine evacuation for gestational trophoblastic disease.

■ Consultation

Figure 4.1 outlines the stages of a consultation for a patient asking for EC. These stages will be explored in more detail as we move through the chapter.

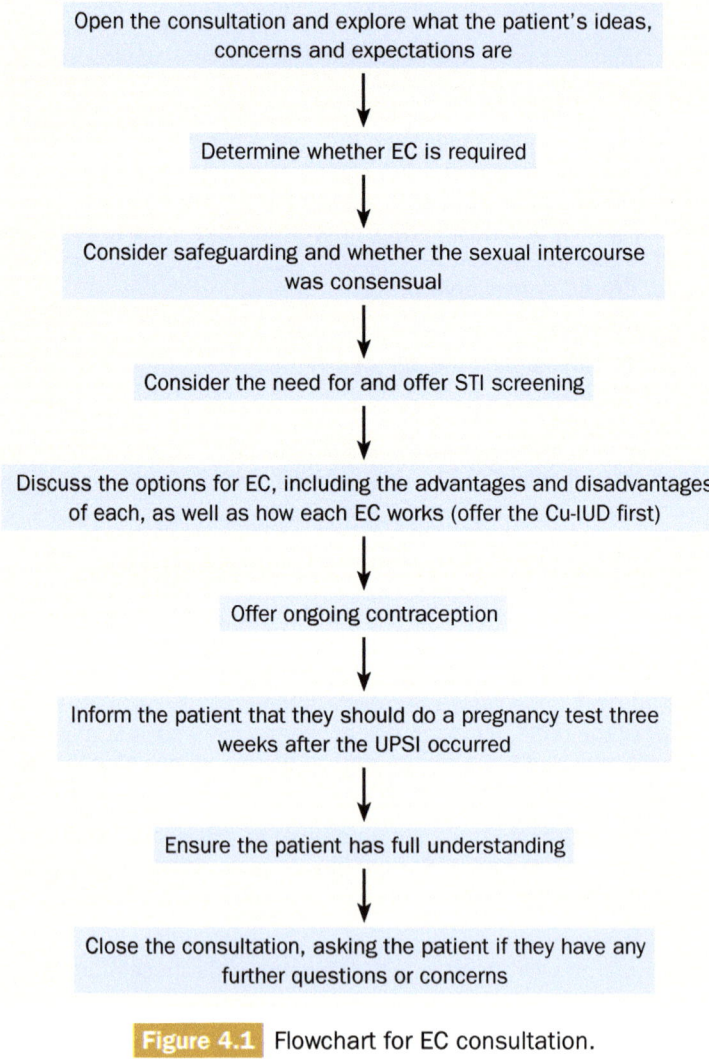

Figure 4.1 Flowchart for EC consultation.

CHAPTER 4 • Emergency Contraception

■ History

During the history-taking phase of the consultation, consider patients' thoughts and feelings and ask the following questions.

- When did the UPSI take place?
- Has there been further episodes of UPSI during this cycle? If so, when and how many times?
- Was the sexual intercourse with a new or regular partner?
- Was the sexual intercourse consensual?
- Have there been multiple partners?
- Is the patient involved in high-risk sexual activity, such as with MSM, or sexual contact with someone from a country with a high prevalence of HIV?

For more on HIV see pp. 95–99 in Chapter 7: Sexually Transmitted Infections and p. 8 in Chapter 1: Communication.

- When was their LMP?
  - Was it a normal period for them?
- Where are they in their current cycle?
  - Sometimes women are unsure about this as they have irregular periods, or they have been taking a hormonal method of contraception and they have not had a period for some time. Other times, patients have recorded their cycle in an app and can clearly tell you the date of their LMP.
- Was any other contraception used or was there a contraception failure (for example, condom splitting, missed pills or late starting a contraceptive method)?
- If they are not currently taking any contraception, would they like ongoing contraception?
- Ask about their thoughts and feelings about the prospect of being pregnant.
- Have they shared their situation with anyone else?
- Where appropriate, consider the patient's age and the age of their partner.

■ Consideration of STIs

When consulting with any female regarding EC, you must consider the risk of an STI and offer screening after taking a comprehensive sexual history.

See Chapter 7: Sexually Transmitted Infections (pp. 85–102).

■ Examination

Other than to measure the patient's BMI in certain circumstances, an examination is not usually required.

43

■ Safeguarding

> As part of your consultation, it is essential that you explore the potential for sexual or domestic abuse. You should always clarify if the sex was with a regular partner, and whether it was consensual and without violence. It is important to ask the patient if they feel safe and happy in their relationship(s) and ensure that the principles of confidentiality are understood insofar as when confidentiality cannot be maintained, for example when a crime has taken place.

If a disclosure is made to you during the consultation regarding sexual crime or violence, the following approach will enable you to support the patient as you navigate your local safeguarding procedures (Luby, 2018).

1. Support the disclosure.
   - Provide a quiet and confidential space for the patient to continue the conversation. Acknowledge that it may be difficult to speak about what happened.
   - Provide an interpreter if English is not the person's first language (do not use a family member or friend).
   - Be non-judgemental, supportive and empathetic.
2. Ensure any medical treatment is provided as a priority.
   - This may require assessment at the emergency department (ED), depending on the injury.
3. Ask the patient what they want to happen next.
   - Inform the patient that they can access an independent domestic and sexual violence advisor (IDSVA) who can help them better understand their options. It is helpful to know how these can be accessed in your local area; it may be via your service, victim support, the police, rape crisis centres, Sexual Assault Referral Centre (SARC) or third sector services. The role of the IDSVA is to provide information and support particularly around the criminal justice process, liaise with work or educational settings and provide therapeutic input.
4. Arrange for police involvement if the patient consents to this, and find the nearest SARC if they have been sexually assaulted.
5. Ensure that sexual health/medical needs are accounted for.
   - EC (unless it is too late, in which case ensure you offer pregnancy testing on the first day of the missed period).
   - If indicated, arrange for post-exposure prophylaxis (PEP) to be prescribed.
   - Hepatitis B vaccination may also be indicated. In some situations, the patient will also need a hepatitis B immunoglobin (HBIG) injection along with the hepatitis B vaccine. This should ideally be given within 48 hours but can still be given up until a week after exposure.
   - Assess the wish or need for referral for further assessment and screening, particularly for STIs; this is usually two weeks after possible exposure.
6. Ensure accurate documentation.

CHAPTER 4 · Emergency Contraception

 For further information, cross-reference with Chapter 8: Safeguarding (pp. 103–122).

■ What Methods of Emergency Contraception are Available?

In the UK, three methods of EC are currently available: Cu-IUD, oral ulipristal acetate (UPA) and oral levonorgestrel (LNG).

Copper IUD

The emergency Cu-IUD works by stopping an egg being fertilised or implanting in the uterus. It is toxic to sperm and eggs and therefore prevents implantation. It is ten times more effective than oral EC (FPA, 2020) and is therefore seen as the gold-standard method of EC.

Ulipristal acetate

This emergency contraceptive pill works by stopping/delaying ovulation, so it is only likely to work if taken before the egg has been released. It is effective up to 120 hours after UPSI. A brand commonly seen in practice is ellaOne® (Figure 4.2).

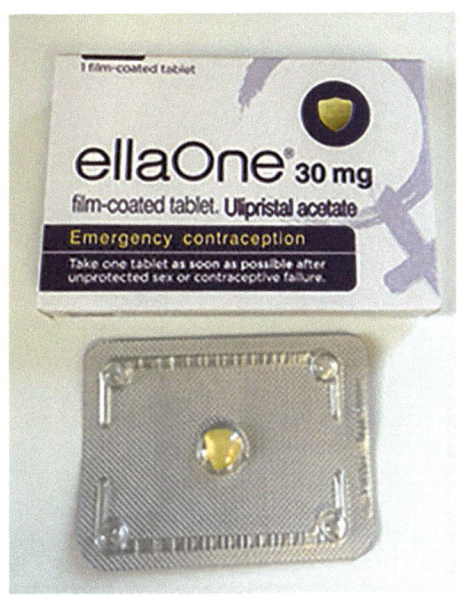

Figure 4.2 ellaOne.

45

Levonorgestrel

This emergency contraceptive pill works by stopping ovulation, so it is only likely to work if taken before the egg has been released. LNG is licensed for use up to 72 hours after UPSI and has reduced efficacy 96 hours after UPSI. A brand commonly seen in practice is Levonelle® (Figure 4.3).

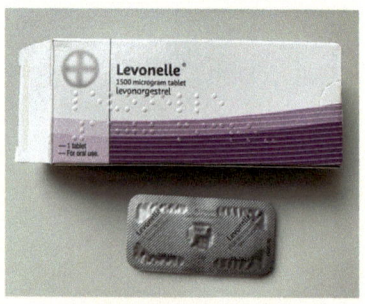

Figure 4.3 Levonelle.

■ Choosing the Most Appropriate Method of Emergency Contraception

 Evidence suggests that the oral EC pills (both LNG and UPA) do not disrupt an existing pregnancy and are not associated with fetal abnormality (FSRH, 2020b).

The National Institute for Health and Care Excellence (Joint Formulary Committee, 2023a) recommends that women who ask for EC should be told that a Cu-IUD is more effective than an oral EC method and this should be offered first. However, you should have an open discussion with the patient and identify which EC option would be most appropriate for them, using the FSRH (2020b) guidance to aid decision making. Remind women that they may still become pregnant, despite taking the EC pill correctly.

 If a woman is referred to have a Cu-IUD inserted then she should be given the EC pill at the time of referral, in case the Cu-IUD cannot be inserted or the woman changes her mind about the form of EC used.

If you are able to prescribe, it is important to know that enzyme-inducing drugs reduce the effects of both LNG and UPA. Women requiring EC who are using enzyme-inducing drugs should be offered the Cu-IUD if appropriate. A double dose of LNG can be considered but the effectiveness of this is unknown. However, a double dose of UPA is not recommended.

A double dose of LNG should be given to women who are over 70 kg (FSRH, 2019b) (therefore it is vital to ask or take their weight), as a higher BMI reduces the effects of LNG.

CHAPTER 4 • Emergency Contraception

The effectiveness of UPA is reduced if a woman takes progestogen in the five days after taking UPA. Additionally, the effectiveness of UPA could be theoretically reduced if a woman has taken progestogen in the seven days before (for example, she had missed a pill). A woman can start her ongoing contraception five days after taking the UPA. This may not be suitable for women who are young and/or those at high risk of becoming pregnant, and therefore LNG may be considered instead.

Table 4.1 summarises the mode of action, advantages, disadvantages, risks, cautions and contraindications for each of the three EC methods.

Table 4.1 Comparison of EC methods.

	Cu-IUD	UPA	LNG
Mode of action	Plastic and copper IUD. An inhibitory effect on both fertilisation and implantation.	Delays ovulation for five days or more.	Inhibits ovulation and causes luteal dysfunction.
Advantages	Highly effective in preventing pregnancy; the most effective method of EC with a failure rate of 1 in 1,000. Non-hormonal. Can be used as ongoing, regular contraception for up to 10 years. Can be inserted up to five days following UPSI.	No long-term side-effects. No procedure needed. Can be taken up to five days after UPSI.	No long-term side-effects. No procedure needed.
Disadvantages	A minor surgical procedure is needed to fit the Cu-IUD. Period-type pain and bleeding are common a few days following insertion. Women will need to be given the EC pill in the interim anyway, as it may not be possible to fit it straight away.	Less effective than the Cu-IUD. May affect the next period. Cannot be taken within five days of taking progestogen (for example, POP). Potential side effects: vomiting and headaches.	Can only be taken up to three days after UPSI. May affect the next period. Less effective than other emergency contraceptive methods. Potential side-effects: vomiting and headaches.

(Continued)

Table 4.1 *(Continued)*

	Cu-IUD	UPA	LNG
Risks	Small risk of infection after insertion. Ascending pelvic infection in women with existing bacterial STI; risk is highest in women with chlamydia or gonorrhoea (BASHH, 2019b). All women requesting Cu-IUD insertion should be individually assessed regarding risk of STIs (FSRH, 2019c). Perforation (up to 2 per 1,000). Expulsion (1 in 20). Ectopic pregnancy, although the overall risk of ectopic pregnancy is reduced with Cu-IUD compared to using no contraception (FSRH, 2023a).		
Cautions		Use with caution in those with severe asthma, controlled by oral glucocorticoids.	Use with caution in those with a BMI of more than 26 or a weight of more than 70 kg.
Contraindications	Less than 28 days following giving birth. Less than five days following a miscarriage or abortion. Active STI.	Less than 21 days following giving birth. Less than five days following a miscarriage or abortion.	Less than 21 days following giving birth. Less than five days following a miscarriage or abortion.

Source: Adapted from Mason (2020).

CHAPTER 4 • Emergency Contraception

Cu-IUD users should be informed about symptoms of ectopic pregnancy. The possibility of ectopic pregnancy should be considered in women with a Cu-IUD who present with abdominal pain, especially in connection with missed periods, or if an amenorrhoeic woman starts bleeding. If a pregnancy test is positive, a USS is urgently required to locate the pregnancy.

The information in Table 4.1 can be relayed to the patient to help them make an informed decision on the most suitable EC method. Further discussion and education on the Cu-IUD such as that listed below has been shown to enhance the likelihood of uptake for this method.

- Using visual aids and models that demonstrate the size of the Cu-IUD.
- Advising women of the high efficacy rate and option for use as an ongoing, long-term method of contraception (Bharadwaj et al., 2011).

Additionally, use the algorithms available for HCPs from the FSRH *Clinical Guideline: Emergency Contraception* (2020b). Figure 4.4 outlines the decision-making process for oral EC (Algorithm 2).

Algorithm 1, found in FSRH (2020b, p. ix of guideline), displays the decision-making process when considering EC: Cu-IUD versus oral EC.

Check to see if there is a coil-fitting clinician available in your surgery to fit an emergency Cu-IUD, which may prevent unnecessary travel for the patient to the nearest genitourinary clinic.

■ Regular Use of Emergency Contraception

If a woman has already taken UPA once or more in a cycle, then she can have UPA again after further UPSI in the same cycle. The same can be said for LNG. However, if a woman has already taken UPA, LNG should not be taken in the following five days. Additionally, if a woman has already taken LNG in her cycle, UPA may be less effective if taken in the following seven days.

■ Emergency Contraception and Transgender Individuals

Trans men and non-binary (assigned female) people who do not wish to become pregnant should be offered EC after unprotected vaginal intercourse

49

Sexual Health and Contraception

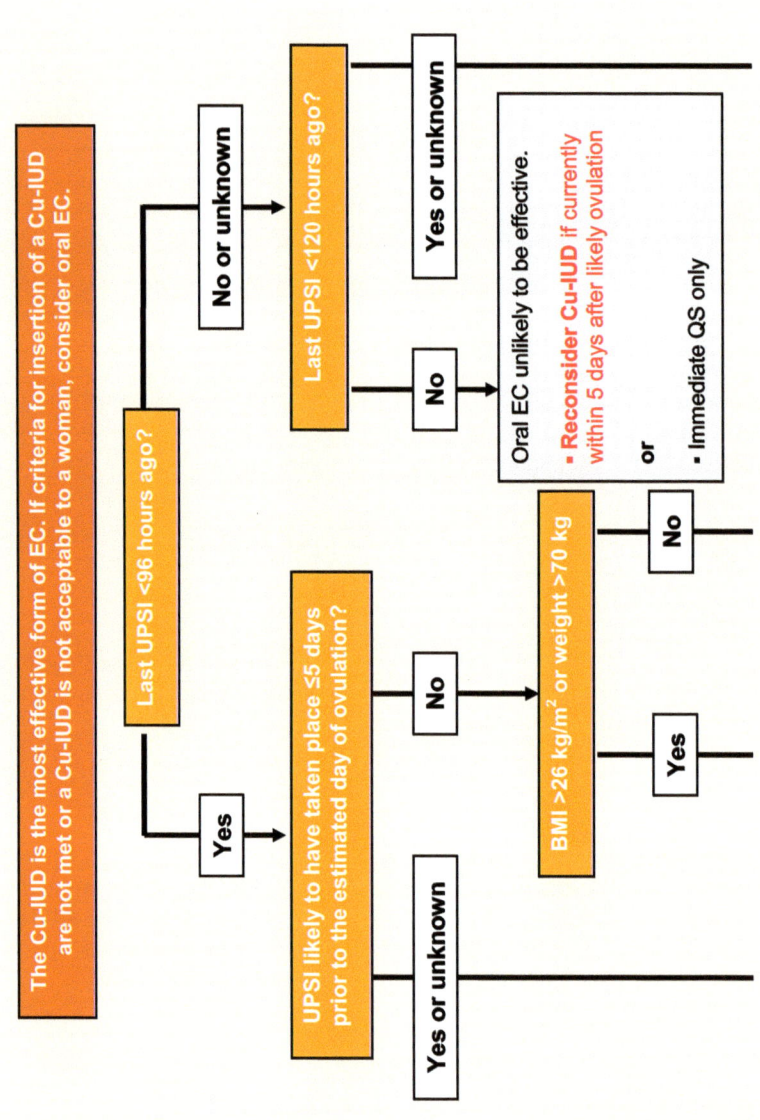

CHAPTER 4 • Emergency Contraception

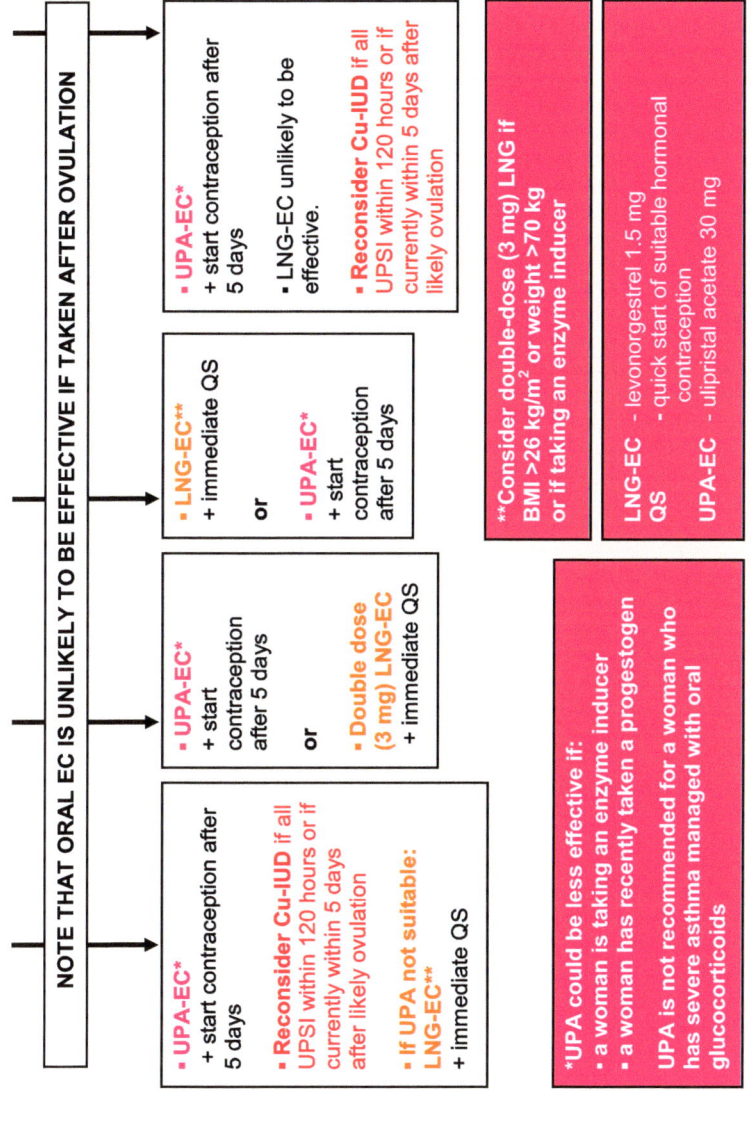

Figure 4.4 Decision-making algorithm for oral EC: LNG versus UPA (Algorithm 2).
Source: FSRH, 2020b.

or if their regular contraception has been compromised or used incorrectly. Both oral EC methods (UPA 30 mg and LNG 1.5 mg) and the Cu-IUD can be used by trans men and non-binary people without interfering with hormone regimens. Testosterone is not thought to affect the efficacy of hormonal EC (FSRH, 2017). Trans men and non-binary people should be informed that the Cu-IUD is the most effective method of EC. Trans men who choose to use oral EC should be informed that these methods do not provide contraceptive cover for subsequent UPSI and that they will need to use contraception or abstain from sexual intercourse to avoid further risk of pregnancy.

Emergency Contraception and Breastfeeding

If the woman is not exclusively breastfeeding but she is still breastfeeding (perhaps alongside formula milk) and/or the baby is not under six months and/or she has had a period, and she requires EC, further precautions need to be taken. Breastfeeding women have a higher relative risk of uterine perforation during insertion of IUCs than non-breastfeeding women, although the absolute risk of perforation is low. Breastfeeding women should be advised not to breastfeed and to express and discard milk for a week after they have taken UPA. Women who breastfeed should be informed that available limited evidence indicates that LNG has no adverse effects on breastfeeding or on their infants (Joint Formulary Committee, 2023b).

Ongoing Contraception

Women requesting EC should be given information regarding all methods of ongoing contraception and how to access these, as it may be appropriate to 'quick start' opportunistic ongoing contraception to prevent pregnancy. Patients should be reminded that oral methods of EC do not provide contraceptive cover for subsequent UPSI.

Pregnancy Testing

Inform the patient that they should do a pregnancy test three weeks after the UPSI occurred and to contact their primary care provider if it is positive. A 'standard' pregnancy test could rule in or rule out pregnancy with reasonable reliability if undertaken more than 21 days after the last episode of UPSI (FSRH, 2020b).

CHAPTER 4 • Emergency Contraception

CASE STUDY

Presenting complaint

A 32-year-old female presents to you asking for the 'morning after pill'.

History

History of presenting complaint

- She tells you that she is not taking any contraception and that she and her husband normally use condoms, but this time they did not.
- They had UPSI 12 hours ago.
- There have been no additional episodes of UPSI this cycle.
- She is happy in her relationship and the sexual intercourse was consensual.
- She declines STI screening and says she is happily married with no other sexual partners.
- She declines ongoing contraception and says 'I have tried it all before and none of it works for me'.
- She has regular periods and is on day 6 of her cycle.

Past medical/family/drug history

- None, normally fit and well, no regular medicines.

Social history

- She has three children and does not want any more. She works part time as a hairdresser. Non-smoker.

Examination

- Her BMI is 27 (weight over 70 kg).

Diagnosis

- She requires EC.

Management plan

- You offer her the Cu-IUD, but she declines this.
- She has had UPSI within 12 hours (and therefore under 96 hours), she has not been taking any contraception prior (not recently taken progestogen) and does not wish to have any ongoing contraception. She does not take any enzyme inducers or glucocorticoids. Therefore, UPA is most suitable, as it is more effective than LNG, particularly as her weight is over 70 kg.
- As it is within your scope of practice, you prescribe this for her (one tablet) and advise her to take it straight away.
- You advise her that she must do a pregnancy test in three weeks' time.
- You also advise her that if she changes her mind regarding ongoing contraception in the future, she should call the primary care practice. You provide her with a leaflet on contraceptive choices and a link to the Sexwise website.
- You offer her STI screening.

CHAPTER 5

Menstrual-Related Complications

■ Introduction

Menstrual-related complications affect around 25% of women in the UK who are of reproductive age. This results in a negative effect on their physical, psychological and social well-being. Managing 'period problems' is often delayed because of the associated stigma. This leaves women unsupported and can lead to the development of long-term consequences of untreated disease (FSRH, 2018). Therefore, it is vital as an HCP to ensure you make your patient feel comfortable and confident enough to discuss their menstrual related issue with you.

■ Types of Menstrual-Related Complications

- Dysmenorrhoea: painful menstrual periods.
- Menorrhagia: heavy menstrual periods.
- Intermenstrual bleeding (IMB)/problematic bleeding with contraception: periods that do not follow a monthly pattern.
- Amenorrhoea: absence of periods.

> Drugs (such as antipsychotics, which can cause increased prolactin levels) and illicit drug use (in particular cocaine and opiates, which can cause hypogonadism) can cause amenorrhoea (Lania et al., 2019), so always include a drug history when consulting with your patient.

- Problematic bleeding due to contraceptives or presence of an STI: irregular bleeding, spotting, frequent or prolonged bleeding can be a direct result of the contraceptive itself.
- Premenstrual syndrome (PMS): a cyclical disorder of the menstrual cycle whereby the daily functioning of women is affected by emotional and physical symptoms.

Premenstrual dysphoric disorder (PMDD) is similar to PMS but it presents with severe depression, anxiety and irritability in the two weeks before the menstrual cycle begins. PMDD affects around 5% of women and they often require medication to help with the severe symptoms (Pearlstein and Steiner, 2008).

■ History Taking

Some possible questions depending on the menstrual-related issue include the following.

- What is the nature of the bleeding and what impact is it having on the woman's life?
- Is the bleeding irregular?
- What is the woman's normal menstrual cycle (such as length of the cycle and number of days of menstruation) and is there any variation of this pattern?
- Is she up to date with cervical screening?
- Is she on any current contraception and if so, what is it? Is she taking it correctly?
- What are her plans for contraception and planning to conceive?
- Is there any chance of pregnancy?
- Are there any symptoms of stress, depression, weight loss, disturbance of perception of weight or shape, level of exercise and chronic systemic illness?
- What age were her closest female relatives at menarche (first menstrual period)?

Family history of late menarche suggests constitutional delay of puberty.

- Are there any symptoms of menopause (for example, hot flushes or vaginal dryness)?

For further information see pp. 73–74 in Chapter 6: Menopause.

- Is there any relevant medical history, such as endometriosis?
- Has she tried any drug treatments for menorrhagia or dysmenorrhoea?
- Is the bleeding associated with pelvic pain?
- Is it painful to have sex (dyspareunia)?
- Is there any post-coital bleeding?
- Take a full sexual history and investigate the likelihood of an STI.
- Characteristics of the pain, if there is pain, including type of pain, timing and duration, severity and exacerbating and alleviating factors.
- Any abnormal discharge?
- Any family history of menorrhagia or dysmenorrhoea?

CHAPTER 5 • Menstrual-Related Complications

■ Examination

Depending on the history and presenting complaint, examination of the patient with menstrual related issues may involve the following.

- Ensuring the patient is haemodynamically stable (particularly in heavy menstrual bleeding).
- Looking for symptoms suggestive of any underlying pathology, such as hypothyroidism (goitre), coagulation disorders (bruises) or polycystic ovary syndrome (PCOS) (acne, overweight, hirsutism).
- Pregnancy test to exclude pregnancy and ectopic pregnancy. A pregnancy test is indicated for sexually active women using hormonal contraception with problematic bleeding.
- Doing a vaginal swab to investigate for infection.
- Performing an abdominal examination to examine for any masses/fibroids.
- Performing a speculum examination of the cervix if trained to do so. If you are not trained to do speculum examination, then arrange for this to be done by a colleague. If taking contraception, a speculum examination should be performed for women who have problematic bleeding if they have persistent bleeding or a change in bleeding after at least three months of use.
- Arranging a full blood count (FBC) to assess for iron deficiency anaemia.

Iron deficiency anaemia is a strong indicator for heavy menstrual bleeding, and therefore it is important to check FBC.

- Arranging for a thyroid function test (TFT) and test for coagulation disorders where appropriate from the history.
- Measuring height and body weight, and calculating BMI for weight-related causes of amenorrhoea.
- Examining for Turner's syndrome (short stature, web neck, shield chest with widely spaced nipples, wide carrying angle, scoliosis), particularly if a patient is amenorrhoeic.

Turner's syndrome is a genetic condition found only in females. Among other things, it affects typical ovarian development, meaning nearly all girls with Turner's syndrome will be infertile.

- Examining for features of Cushing's syndrome (striae, buffalo hump, significant central obesity, easy bruising, hypertension, proximal muscle weakness).

Menstrual irregularity is a common complaint at presentation in women with Cushing's syndrome.

- Considering arranging a USS to examine for fibroids, adnexal pathology and endometriosis, or to assess positioning of an IUC.

- Considering outpatient hysteroscopy if history is suggestive of submucosal fibroids, polyps or endometrial pathology.
- Offering a transvaginal ultrasound scan (TVUSS) to women with menorrhagia who have significant dysmenorrhoea or a bulky, tender uterus on examination that suggests adenomyosis (where the tissue that normally lines the uterus [endometrial tissue] grows into the muscular wall of the uterus).

A pelvic examination is inappropriate in girls and women who are not/have never been sexually active; a lower abdominal USS can be requested to assess pelvic anatomy.

It is not necessary to measure blood loss to diagnose menorrhagia. Bleeding is considered heavy if it interferes with normal activities (Parker, 2022).

■ Dysmenorrhoea

Diagnosis

Primary dysmenorrhoea (absence of any identifiable underlying pelvic pathology) is the most likely diagnosis when (NICE, 2018a):

- menstrual pain starts 6–12 months after menarche, once cycles are regular
- lower abdominal pain, usually cramping in nature, occurs, which may also radiate to the back and inner thigh
- the pain starts shortly before the onset of menstruation and lasts for up to 72 hours, improving as the period progresses
- non-gynaecological symptoms, such as nausea, vomiting, diarrhoea, fatigue, irritability, dizziness, bloating, headache, lower back pain and emotional symptoms, are often present
- other gynaecological symptoms are not present
- pelvic examination is normal.

Secondary dysmenorrhoea is the most likely diagnosis when (NICE, 2018a):

- the pain starts after several years of painless periods
- it is not consistently related to menstruation alone and may persist after menstruation finishes or may be present throughout the menstrual cycle, but is exacerbated by menstruation
- other gynaecological symptoms, such as dyspareunia, vaginal discharge, menorrhagia, IMB and post-coital bleeding, are often present
- pelvic examination is abnormal, although the absence of abnormal findings does not exclude secondary dysmenorrhoea.

Causes

Secondary causes of dysmenorrhoea include the following (NICE, 2018a).

- Endometriosis/adenomyosis – characterised by cyclical or chronic pelvic pain frequently occurring prior to menstruation and accompanied by heavy menstrual bleeding and deep dyspareunia.

 Rectal pain or bleeding may indicate rectovaginal endometriosis.

- Fibroids may result in lower abdominal pain, frequently accompanied by menorrhagia; a pelvic mass may be identified on examination.
- Pelvic inflammatory disease (PID) which may cause lower abdominal pain and tenderness that may be accompanied by dyspareunia, abnormal vaginal bleeding and abnormal vaginal discharge. In acute infection, fever may be present.
- Ovarian cancer which may cause pelvic or abdominal pain, abdominal distension, loss of appetite and increased urinary urgency and/or frequency. There may be abnormal or postmenopausal bleeding and gastrointestinal symptoms (such as dyspepsia or nausea).
- Cervical cancer is characterised by pelvic pain, dyspareunia, intermenstrual or post-coital bleeding, post-menopausal bleeding and blood-stained, mucoid or purulent vaginal discharge.
- An IUC may be a secondary cause of dysmenorrhoea (usually following insertion 3–6 months previously). Pain may be accompanied by longer and heavier periods, often with IMB or spotting. The IUC may require removal and an alternative form of contraception considered.

Management

Management of primary dysmenorrhoea includes the following.

- Offer an NSAID, unless contraindicated, such as ibuprofen, naproxen or mefenamic acid (refer to the BNF).
- Offer paracetamol if NSAIDs are contraindicated or not tolerated, or in addition if the response is insufficient.
- If the woman does not wish to conceive, consider prescribing a 3–6-month trial of a hormonal contraceptive as an alternative first-line treatment.
- COCP preparations containing 30–35 micrograms of ethinylestradiol (EE) and norethisterone, norgestimate or levonorgestrel are usually first choice, as these are less likely to cause irregular bleeding.
- Progestogen-only contraceptives may also be considered after a full discussion of the advantages and disadvantages, such as the COCP being contraindicated.

 Refer to Chapter 3: Contraception (pp. 19–39) for more detail.

If the response to individual treatments is insufficient, a combination of an NSAID (or paracetamol) and hormonal contraception may be considered.

- The woman may also like to consider non-drug treatments, such as heat or a transcutaneous electrical nerve stimulation (TENS) machine.
- Provide a PIL on dysmenorrhoea.
- If symptoms are severe and do not respond to initial treatment within 3–6 months, or if there is doubt about the diagnosis, referral to a gynaecologist should be considered.

Management of secondary dysmenorrhoea includes the following.

> Suspect a serious secondary cause of dysmenorrhoea and refer urgently if any of the following 'red flags' are present (NICE, 2018a).
> - Ascites
> - Abdominal mass
> - Abnormal cervical examination
> - Persistent IMB or post-coital bleeding
> - A USS suggestive of cancer
> - A raised CA125 blood test.

Consider and manage other causes of secondary dysmenorrhoea such as PID (with antibiotics and in line with BASHH guidelines).

Menorrhagia

Diagnosis

- It is not necessary to measure blood loss to diagnose heavy bleeding.
- Look for features of other underlying disease when assessing a woman with menorrhagia. This should include hypothyroidism, coagulation disorders and PCOS.

Causes

- Hormonal imbalance
- Uterine fibroids
- Polyps
- Adenomyosis
- Contraceptives
- Cancer
- Endometriosis
- PID
- PCOS
- Drugs such as chemotherapy and anticoagulant medicines
- Stress and depression.

CHAPTER 5 • Menstrual-Related Complications

Management

Refer the woman urgently if physical examination identifies ascites and/or a pelvic or abdominal mass.

Refer the woman using a suspected cancer pathway referral (for an appointment within two weeks) if she has a pelvic mass associated with any other features of cancer (such as unexplained bleeding, post-menopausal bleeding or weight loss).

Refer women urgently for suspected cancer if there is post-menopausal bleeding (NICE, 2018b).

HRT and irregular bleeding is detailed on pp. 81–82 in Chapter 6: Menopause.

For more information, see *Gynaecological Cancers – Recognition and Referral* (NICE, 2021b).

Additional reasons warranting referral include the following.
- Women who have complications, such as compressive symptoms from large fibroids (for example dyspareunia, pelvic pain or discomfort, constipation or urinary symptoms).
- If a woman has iron deficiency anaemia which has failed to respond to treatment, and other causes have been excluded, or menorrhagia has not improved despite initial treatments.

Always consider a pregnancy test to rule out ectopic pregnancy where the history is suggestive of this.

Pharmacological treatment such as tranexamic acid and/or an NSAID can be used.

As with dysmenorrhoea, contraceptive methods may help with heavy bleeding, depending on the woman's wishes regarding conception. It is not generally recommended that a contraceptive be changed within the first three months of use, as bleeding disturbances often settle in this time. For women using a COCP, the lowest dose of EE to provide good cycle control should be used. However, the dose of EE can be increased to a maximum of 35 micrograms to provide good cycle control. Bleeding is common in the initial months of using progestogen-only contraceptives (FSRH, 2015).

There is no evidence that changing the type and dose of the POP will improve problematic bleeding; bleeding patterns may vary with different POP preparations and this may help some individuals.

Amenorrhoea

Diagnosis
- Primary amenorrhoea.
  - Absence of periods.
  - Girls who have not established menstruation by the age of 13 years and have no secondary sexual characteristics (such as breast development).
  - Girls who have not established menstruation by the age of 15 years and have normal secondary sexual characteristics.
- Secondary amenorrhoea.
  - Cessation of menstruation for 3–6 months in women with previously normal and regular menses.
  - Cessation of menstruation for 6–12 months in women with previous oligomenorrhoea.

 Oligomenorrhoea is the medical term for infrequent menstrual periods (fewer than 6–8 periods per year).

Causes
- Pregnancy
- Family history
- Diet
- Weight
- Stress
- Contraceptives
- Menopause
- PCOS
- Thyroid disease
- Diabetes
- An extreme exercise pattern
- Turner's syndrome.

Management
Management of primary amenorrhoea includes the following.

- Refer patients with primary amenorrhoea to secondary care for specialist investigation and management of the underlying cause.
- Referral to a gynaecologist is appropriate for most people, but referral to an endocrinologist is recommended for those with hyperprolactinaemia, thyroid disease or features of androgen excess (such as hirsutism or acne).
- Manage amenorrhoea caused by stress, weight loss, excessive exercise or chronic illness after an endocrinologist has assessed and excluded other hypothalamic or pituitary causes (such as a tumour).
- For stress-related amenorrhoea, consider measures to manage stress and improve coping strategies, such as cognitive behavioural therapy (CBT).

CHAPTER 5 • Menstrual-Related Complications

- For weight-related amenorrhoea, encourage weight gain and refer to a dietician. If an eating disorder is suspected, consider referral to specialist services and/or a psychiatrist.
- For exercise-related amenorrhoea, advise reducing exercise, increasing calorie intake and weight gain. Consider referral to, or liaison with, a sports physician or dietician.

You should be particularly aware of eating disorders when dealing with weight loss and exercise-related amenorrhoea. 'Beat Eating Disorders' is a useful resource to support patients with eating disorders. The national helpline can help patients get the support they need.
▶ Search: Beat Eating Disorders.

If amenorrhoea persists for more than 12 months, consider whether osteoporosis prophylaxis is required, but this should be discussed with a primary care provider.

Management of secondary amenorrhoea includes the following. Manage the following causes for secondary amenorrhoea in primary care.

- PCOS, when appropriate.
- Hypothyroidism (menses may take several months to resume with treatment).
- Menopause (women 40 years of age or older).
- Pregnancy.

Refer all other people with secondary amenorrhoea for specialist investigation to a gynaecologist (NICE, 2022b).

■ Problematic Bleeding While Taking Contraception

Problematic bleeding while taking contraception is common and is usually as a result of the contraceptive itself. After reassurance that there is no sinister cause for the bleeding, women are often content to continue their method of contraception.

Before starting contraception, women should always be advised about the possibility of problematic bleeding when using contraceptives (FSRH, 2015). They should be advised that unscheduled bleeding in the first three months after starting a new hormonal contraceptive method is common. This commonly continues to at least six months with the LNG-IUS and progestogen-only implants (FSRH, 2015).

Different contraceptives suit different individuals and finding the correct method for that particular patient can be challenging and take time. For example, the implant may cause prolonged irregular bleeding in some women, but others will be amenorrhoeic. Additionally, adherence to the contraceptive is a common factor for unscheduled bleeding.

Smoking can affect cycle control and therefore encouragement to cease smoking is very important.

For further information regarding the expected bleeding patterns after commencing contraception, see *FSRH Clinical Guideline: Problematic Bleeding with Hormonal Contraception* (FSRH, 2015).

Management

- If bleeding persists after three cycles, consider changing formulation.
- Increase dose of oestrogen, particularly if on a 20 microgram EE preparation, to a maximum of 35 micrograms of EE (there is no evidence that increasing the dose from 30 micrograms to 35 micrograms is effective, but it may work for some women).
- Consider tailored pill regimens.

Tailored regimens information is on p. 30 in Chapter 3: Contraception.

- If bleeding persists despite a different formulation, consider an alternative form of contraception.

Clinicians should follow the FSRH clinical guideline for problematic bleeding with hormonal contraception. Figure 5.1 shows an algorithm to follow when managing women using hormonal contraception who are experiencing problematic bleeding.

If a woman is suffering with IMB but is not on any form of contraception, investigations may include the following (NICE, 2018b).

- FBC, clotting, TFT, FSH/LH blood tests.
- Pregnancy test.
- Cervical screening if it is due.
- STI screening.
- Examination of the cervix. If there is a concerning appearance of the cervix then refer urgently for suspected cancer.
- Consider TVUSS if persistent.
- If the TVUSS is normal then consider methods to regulate the cycle, such as the COCP.
- There should be a low threshold to refer women with persistent irregular bleeding, especially if they are obese or have PCOS, due to a higher risk of endometrial pathology.
- Refer women urgently to a gynaecology clinic if they are 40 years of age or over with persistent IMB (>3 consecutive months who are not using hormonal contraceptives) and no concerning appearances of the cervix. Also refer for urgent TVUSS at the time of referral.

CHAPTER 5 • Menstrual-Related Complications

 Women should be reassured that IMB is common and symptoms often spontaneously resolve and that underlying cancer is rare.

Premenstrual Syndrome

PMS describes a wide variety of physical and psychological symptoms associated with the menstrual cycle. About 30–40% of women experience symptoms severe enough to disrupt their daily lives. PMS symptoms are more severe and disruptive than the typical mild premenstrual symptoms that as many as 75% of all women experience (Parker, 2022). It is caused by rising and falling levels of oestrogen and progesterone, which may influence certain brain chemicals, including serotonin, though it is not clear why some women develop PMS (Parker, 2022).

Physical symptoms associated with PMS include:
- bloating
- swollen, painful breasts
- fatigue
- constipation
- headaches
- 'clumsiness'.

Emotional symptoms associated with PMS include:
- anger
- anxiety or confusion
- mood swings and tension
- crying and depression
- inability to concentrate.

Diagnosis
- Ask the woman to record a daily symptom diary for two or three cycles, and review the woman with the diary.

 The Daily Record of Severity of Problems (DRSP) is a validated questionnaire that is widely used for tracking symptoms related to PMS.

- Diagnose PMS if the symptom diary shows prominence of symptoms during the luteal phase of the menstrual cycle, which resolve with the onset of menses or soon after, followed by a symptom-free week.
- Symptoms should be severe enough to affect daily functioning (consider PMDD if very severe symptoms).
- If cyclical symptoms are not found, exclude other conditions that could explain the symptoms, such as depression and peri-menopause (NICE, 2019a).

- Take a clinical history to assess:
  - The woman's concerns
  - Correct use of method (e.g. pill taking, patch use), use of interacting medication, illness altering absorption of orally administered hormones
  - Other symptoms (e.g. pain, dyspareunia, abnormal vaginal discharge, heavy bleeding, post-coital bleeding)
- Exclude sexually transmitted infections
- Check cervical screening history
- Consider the need for a pregnancy test

↓

Manage any issues identified above

↓ ↓

Less than 3 months since starting the method: [a]

All of the above checked and confirmed/excluded. Thereafter a gynaecological examination and further investigation (biopsy, scan, hysteroscopy) are not routinely required

Reassure and arrange follow-up

If requested, medical management can be considered

NB: LNG-IUS users with pain, discharge or non-visible threads in addition to bleeding require investigation to exclude expulsion, perforation or infection

[a] 3 months is an arbitrary cut-off and is not evidence based. Persistent bleeding is common in the first 6 months of use with LNG-IUS and progestogen-only implants

More than 3 months use with: [a]
- Persistent bleeding
- New symptoms or changed bleeding pattern
- Failed medical treatment
- Not participating in a cervical screening programme
- If requested by the woman

[a] 3 months is an arbitrary cut-off and is not evidence based. Persistent bleeding is common in the first 6 months of use with LNG-IUS and progestogen-only implants

CHAPTER 5 • Menstrual-Related Complications

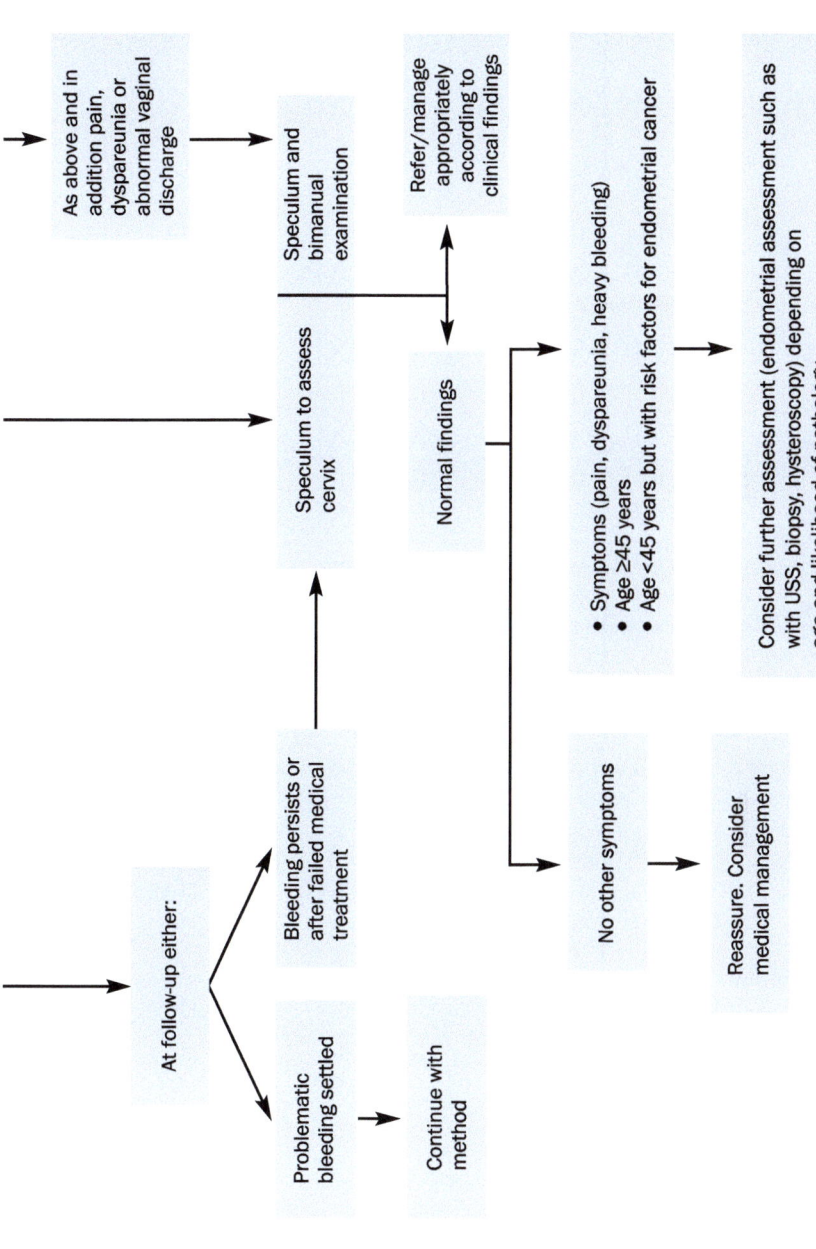

Figure 5.1 Algorithm for the management of women on hormonal contraception experiencing problematic bleeding. *Source*: FSRH, 2015.

Management

Management of PMS should be tailored to the severity and type of symptoms, the woman's treatment preferences and any desire to become pregnant.

Offer lifestyle advice that includes:
- regular, frequent (2–3 hourly), small, balanced meals rich in complex carbohydrates
- regular exercise
- regular sleep
- stress reduction
- smoking and/or vaping cessation (if applicable)
- alcohol restriction (if applicable)
- offering pain relief, if the predominant symptom is pain.

There is a significant link between dietary habits and lifestyle factors (smoking and alcohol) and PMS, therefore promotion of a healthy lifestyle is key for these patients (Hashim et al., 2019).

- Provide a PIL.
- Consider prescribing a COCP, especially if the woman requires contraception. Current data suggest use of the COCP continuously rather than cyclically. Advise the woman that it is not possible to predict whether PMS symptoms will respond to the treatment.
- Arrange referral for CBT if it is thought that the woman would benefit from psychological intervention.
- Only if severe, consider prescribing a selective serotonin reuptake inhibitor (SSRI) (off-label use) to be taken continuously or just during the luteal phase (for example, days 15–28 of the menstrual cycle). In people younger than 18 years of age, prescribe an SSRI only on the advice of a specialist. Do not prescribe an SSRI if there is doubt about the diagnosis or a lack of experience in prescribing them. This will probably need to be discussed with a primary care provider (NICE, 2019a).

CASE STUDY

Presenting complaint

You are working at a walk-in-centre and a 19-year-old female patient presents to you complaining of irregular bleeding.

History

History of presenting complaint

- She tells you that she started the POP two months ago and the irregular bleeding has been since then.
- She tells you that there have been no missed pills.

CHAPTER 5 • Menstrual-Related Complications

- She is not sexually active; she started the POP because she wanted to stop her periods completely, as she is a swimmer.
- She is not pregnant.
- She suffers with migraines with aura and therefore the COCP is contraindicated.
- You discussed all options for contraception at the initial consultation when she commenced on the POP, and she was adamant she did not want the coil, injection or implant.
- She feels well in herself, no dizziness.
- She describes the bleeding as light but 'annoying'.
- No abdominal pain.
- Her mood is good, other than being frustrated with the bleeding – it occurs almost daily.

Past medical history
None.

Social/family/drug history
- She has no significant relevant family history.
- She drinks a moderate amount of alcohol at the weekend, does not take drugs and is a non-smoker.

Examination
- She appears well.
- Her blood pressure is 122/82.
- Her BMI is 24.
- No abdominal masses.

Preferred diagnosis
The irregular bleeding is most likely due to the POP.

Management plan
- You suggest that as this issue has arisen since she started the POP, then this is probably the cause.
- You advise her that it is very common to get irregular bleeding on the POP, particularly in the first three months.
- You revisit the alternative options of contraception, but she would rather persevere with the POP.
- You do not feel it is necessary to do a pregnancy test since she has never been sexually active.
- It is not necessary to do a speculum examination at this point.
- You advise her to call back if the bleeding gets heavier or is associated with any pain, or if it is not settling after three months.
- You also advise her that the POP may not completely stop her bleeding.
- Remind her that the POP does not protect her from STIs.

69

CHAPTER 6

Menopause

■ Introduction

The menopause is typically determined as two years after last having a period if the patient is under the age of 50 and one year if they are over 50 (FPA, 2020). Seventy-five percent of menopausal women have symptoms and one-third of these women have severe symptoms that can last for many years (Hamoda et al., 2016). In 2017, the British Menopause Society (BMS) reported on a nationally representative online survey conducted on their behalf with 1,000 adults in the UK (698 women and 302 men) who were aged 45+ and either peri-menopausal, menopausal or post-menopausal or partners of those who were. The symptoms women described included hot flushes, night sweats and low levels of energy. Three-quarters of the women said that the menopause had strongly affected aspects of their lives and more than half said it had had a negative impact on their lives. The findings of this study are highlighted in Figure 6.1. A third of the women surveyed were experiencing symptoms but had not tried anything to reduce or prevent them, even when all aspects of their lives were affected, including their relationships. The findings of the survey suggest that menopause remains a 'taboo' subject in the UK, something that women and men are not comfortable talking about (BMS, 2020).

Recommendations in the NICE guideline: *Menopause: Diagnosis and Management* (2019b) begin by reminding us of the importance of acknowledging a patient's individuality and the unique way in which the menopause might be having an impact on their social and working life. An individualised approach is recommended which includes avoiding pathologising the menopause. Some women might welcome a conversation that sees menopause purely as a 'hormonal deficiency' that can be addressed with HRT (Menopause Charity, 2021). Others, in contrast, might need to talk about how they are feeling in relation to ageing and the changes happening in their lives. We should not underestimate the influences of societal pressures and conditioning which may be having an impact on a woman's sexuality and self-esteem.

In past decades, the use of HRT for menopausal women has raised criticism and alarm. This chapter offers an opportunity to review changes in opinion due

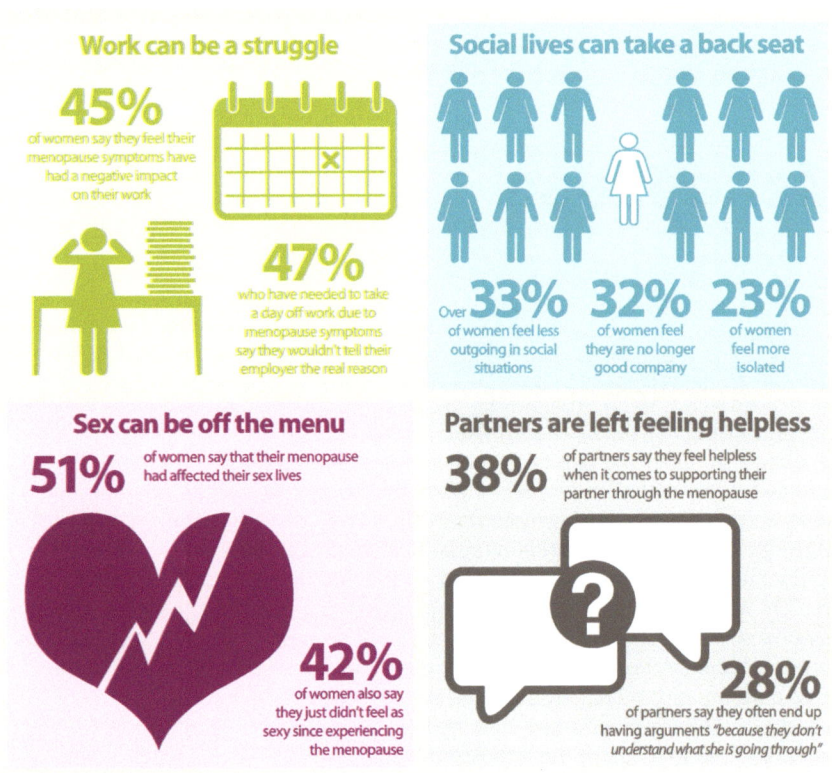

Figure 6.1 Statistics related to the menopause.
Source: BMS (2020). Reproduced with permission.

to recent research evidence demonstrating the benefits of HRT in terms of symptom relief as well as long-term health outcomes.

In a survey of primary care providers with interest in the menopause, 92% felt they were well placed to manage menopause in primary care (Newson and Mair, 2018); however, only 40% of these providers had attended formal menopause training. A lack of knowledge and understanding of the menopause can lead to unnecessary tests and investigations. This might include inappropriate referrals – for example, rheumatology for aching joints and muscles; cardiology for palpitations; headache clinic for an increase in headaches and migraines; memory clinic for forgetfulness; and cystoscopies for recurrent UTIs. It is not just HCPs who can miss linking symptoms to the menopause. Studies consistently show that many women are not aware that their symptoms are menopause related.

Primary care practitioners are in an ideal position to adopt a holistic approach to menopause, one that considers enhancing health and well-being whilst considering an individual's needs, preferences and values. The key principles that should underpin menopause service provision are outlined on the website of the BMS (2020). This includes the following recommendations.

- All HCPs should have a basic understanding of the menopause and know where to signpost women for advice, support and treatment whenever appropriate.
- Every primary care team should have at least one nominated HCP with a special interest in and knowledge of menopause.
- All HCPs with a special interest in menopause should have access to BMS menopause specialists for advice, support, onward referral and leadership of multidisciplinary education.

It is worth remembering that anyone with a female reproductive system who identifies as a man or as non-binary but has not undergone any medical interventions is likely to go through the menopause eventually. If a trans person starts hormonal transition treatment at a premenopausal age, they will not experience the hormone depletion associated with the menopause since gender-affirming hormones are typically given for life.

■ Definitions of Menopause and Peri-Menopause

- Menopause marks the end of the menstrual cycle when ovaries have stopped functioning.
    - Clinical definition: one year and a day since last menstrual period.
    - Average age: 51.
    - Age range: 45–55.
- Peri-menopause: the period leading up to menopause – can be 10 years of hormone fluctuations.
- Early menopause.
    - Age: <45
    - Prevalence: 1 in 10.
- Premature ovarian insufficiency (POI).
    - Age: <40.
    - Prevalence: 1 in 100.
    - This can occur naturally or be induced (for example, following a hysterectomy and/or oophorectomy or some cancer treatments).

■ Common Presenting Symptoms

Women present with a range of symptoms associated with the menopause. These are due to a reduction in oestrogen and include the following.

- Vasomotor: hot flushes, night sweats.

- Genitourinary: vaginal dryness, itching, soreness, urinary frequency, incontinence, increased tendency for UTIs.
- Menstrual: changes to pattern and/or heavier/lighter periods.
- Emotional: low mood, depression, anxiety, worsening PMS.
- Others: poor sleep, tiredness, joint and muscle pain, headaches, migraines, lack of libido, skin changes, hair thinning, palpitations, difficulty concentrating, brain fog, increased weight and body shape changes.

Women can be encouraged to use a symptom questionnaire to identify their profile of menopausal symptoms such as the one from Balance (Table 6.1). This can be used to monitor symptoms and is worth doing regularly to assess how symptoms change with time or treatment.

Making a Diagnosis

As identified in the NICE guideline *Menopause: Diagnosis and Management* (2019b), laboratory tests should not be used as diagnostic tools in otherwise healthy women aged over 45 years with menopausal symptoms. To avoid costly and unnecessary FSH testing, the presence of the following three factors can be used to provide an adequate diagnosis of peri-menopause/menopause.

- Peri-menopause based on vasomotor symptoms and irregular periods.
- Menopause in women who have not had a period for over 12 months and are not using hormonal contraception.
- Menopause based on symptoms in women without a uterus.

Follicle-stimulating hormone testing

Consider using an FSH test to diagnose menopause only:

- in women aged 40–45 years with menopausal symptoms, including a change in their menstrual cycle
- in women aged under 40 years in whom menopause is suspected.

In these cases, it is suggested two readings are taken, six weeks apart. Occasionally, these results will be normal, in which case a clinical diagnosis, based on symptoms, is acceptable.

Testing FSH levels can be effective for women with an IUS or on the POP; however, the combined hormonal contraceptive pill should be stopped at least six weeks prior to testing, in order to obtain an accurate result.

Undertaking a TFT to exclude hypothyroidism as a cause of fatigue should be considered.

Table 6.1 Menopause Symptom Questionnaire©.

Symptoms	Not at all 0	A little 1	Quite a bit 2	Extremely 3	Comment
Heart beating quickly or strongly					
Feeling tense or nervous					
Difficulty in sleeping					
Memory problems					
Attacks of anxiety, panic					
Difficulty in concentrating					
Feeling tired or lacking in energy					
Loss of interest in most things					
Feeling unhappy or depressed					
Crying spells					
Irritability					
Feeling dizzy or faint					
Pressure or tightness in head					
Tinnitus (ringing or buzzing in the ear)					
Headaches					
Muscle and joint pains					
Pins and needles in any part of the body					
Breathing difficulties					
Hot flushes					
Sweating at night					
Loss of interest in sex					
Urinary symptoms					
Symptoms due to vaginal dryness					
SCORE:					

Source: Newson (2021). Reproduced with the kind permission of Balance. Originally created by Dr Louise Newson.

Diagnosing premature ovarian insufficiency

As many as 1 in 100 women under the age of 40 in the UK will experience POI (Daisy Network, 2023). A diagnosis of POI can be based on menopausal symptoms, including absent or infrequent periods for four months and two elevated FSH levels (>25 IU/l) taken 4–6 weeks apart.

Women with a potential or actual diagnosis of POI should be referred to a specialist with expertise in this condition. Hormonal treatment of POI is important to prevent associated longer term health sequalae (NICE, 2022c).

For more information on POI visit the Daisy Network (2023).

■ Information Sharing and Advice

Conversations with individuals about the menopause should always be seen as information sharing rather than a one-way process of providing information. It is important that women are given the opportunity to discuss their symptoms and ideas about potential management. NICE (2022c) identifies the importance of including family members or carers where appropriate. Topics for discussion are:

- an explanation of the stages of menopause
- common symptoms and diagnosis
- lifestyle changes and interventions that could help general health and well-being
- benefits and risks of treatments for menopausal symptoms
- long-term health implications of menopause.

The following types of treatment for menopause symptoms can be discussed.

- Hormonal, for example, HRT.
- Non-hormonal, for example, clonidine.
- Non-pharmaceutical, for example, CBT.

It important to remember that women in the peri-menopausal and early menopausal stages can be at risk of pregnancy and it is therefore necessary to undertake a pregnancy test and discuss contraception where appropriate (FSRH, 2019a).

Resources for service users are provided on p. 83.

■ Managing the Menopause

Table 6.2 presents a summary of the management of menopausal symptoms.

Table 6.2 Management of menopausal symptoms.

Symptoms	Management	Additional considerations
Vasomotor symptoms	Offer HRT after discussing short- and long-term benefits and risks: • oestrogen and progestogen to women with a uterus • oestrogen alone to women without a uterus. See *HRT–Practical Prescribing* (Stephens et al., 2021).	Do not offer SSRIs or SNRIs (serotonin–norepinephrine reuptake inhibitor) or clonidine as first-line treatment. Some evidence that plant-based remedies such as isoflavones or black cohosh may relieve symptoms (safety uncertain; different preparations may vary; interactions with other medicines have been reported).
Psychological symptoms	Consider HRT to alleviate low mood as a result of menopause. Consider CBT to alleviate low mood or anxiety as a result of menopause.	No clear evidence for SSRIs or SNRIs to ease low mood in menopausal women who have not been diagnosed with depression.
Altered sexual function	Consider testosterone supplementation for menopausal women with low sexual desire if HRT alone is not effective.	Testosterone is off-label use.
Urogenital atrophy	Offer vaginal oestrogen (including women on systemic HRT). Consider vaginal oestrogen when systemic HRT is contraindicated after seeking advice from an HCP with expertise in menopause. Water-based vaginal lubricant for sexual activity.	See Position Statement for Management of genitourinary syndrome of the menopause (GSM) (British Society for Sexual Medicine, 2023).

Source: NICE (2022c).

Hormone Replacement Therapy

When discussing HRT treatment options, there is often confusion between 'body-identical HRT' and 'bio-identical HRT'.

- Body-identical HRT includes transdermal oestrogen and micronised progesterone – they are molecularly identical to hormones produced in the ovaries. These are regulated and authorised treatments.
- Bio-identical HRT (compounded bio-identical) hormones: this form of HRT is often provided by private practitioners and is very expensive. The products are not regulated or licensed and therefore caution is needed due to unknown efficacy and safety.

Benefits and risks of hormone replacement therapy

There is general agreement on some of the key benefits of HRT but different opinions and interpretations of the risks are still prevalent and are often based on myths and misconceptions. It is sometimes worth explaining the flaws in a large early study of HRT: the Women's Health Initiative study (WHI, 2002). This study included women who were postmenopausal, overweight, had a history of cardiovascular disease (CVD) and were also prescribed synthetic HRT. Subsequent revised data from this study and the findings of more recent randomised controlled trials have provided more robust evidence to inform clinical decision making as identified in the textbook, *Managing the Menopause: 21st century solutions* (Panay et al., 2015). This evidence suggests that HRT should be offered to well-informed peri-menopausal or early postmenopausal women in order to control moderate to severe menopausal symptoms.

Any discussion about the benefits and risks of HRT should also include the long-term health risks that are associated with the menopause itself due to a reduction in oestrogen.

- CVD is the most common cause of mortality in women worldwide, accounting for 45% of total mortality, with a significant increase in risk after the menopause.

All peri-menopausal women who seek help to control menopausal symptoms should be evaluated for the risk of developing CVD – namely high blood pressure, central obesity, dyslipidaemia and impaired glucose tolerance, and specifically women with a family history of CVD.

- Osteoporosis: bone density decreases after menopause; one in two women will have a fracture over 50 years of age.

Benefits of hormone replacement therapy

For healthy menopausal women below the age of 60, with troublesome symptoms, the benefits of HRT for symptom control or alleviation outweigh the risks as shown in Table 6.3.

Risks of hormone replacement therapy

The risks associated with HRT are usually very small and depend on the type of HRT, the length of time for which it is taken and individual health risks.

Table 6.3 Benefits of HRT for menopausal symptom control.

Menopause-associated symptoms	Alleviation with HRT
Vasomotor	Consensus statements and the NICE menopause guideline (2022c) recommend the use of HRT for vasomotor symptoms.
CVD risk	Cochrane analysis suggests that HRT (oestrogen with or without progestogen) started before the age of 60 years or within ten years of the menopause is associated with a reduction in atherosclerosis progression, coronary heart disease and death from cardiovascular causes as well as all-cause mortality (Hillard et al., 2021).
Osteoporosis	HRT has been shown to be effective in preserving bone density, preventing osteoporosis and reducing osteoporosis-related fractures in both spine and hip (Hillard et al., 2021).
Genitourinary syndrome	Topical HRT can be effective without the need for systemic HRT (Hamoda et al., 2016).
Emotional	Both combined and oestrogen-only preparations improve low mood, anxiety and depressive symptoms.

This overview of evidence about the risks of HRT is based on the NHS website for service users, which provides a simplified overview (NHS, 2022b).

Breast cancer

Combined HRT can be associated with a small increased risk of breast cancer. The increased risk is related to how long HRT is taken for and falls after treatment is stopped.

The importance of breast awareness and attending breast cancer screening should be discussed with women taking HRT.

Figure 6.2 highlights the risks of breast cancer and can be helpful to share with women to aid decision making.

Venous thromboembolism risk

- No increased risk from transdermal HRT (patches, gels or sprays).
- A small increased VTE risk from oral HRT preparations.

Sexual Health and Contraception

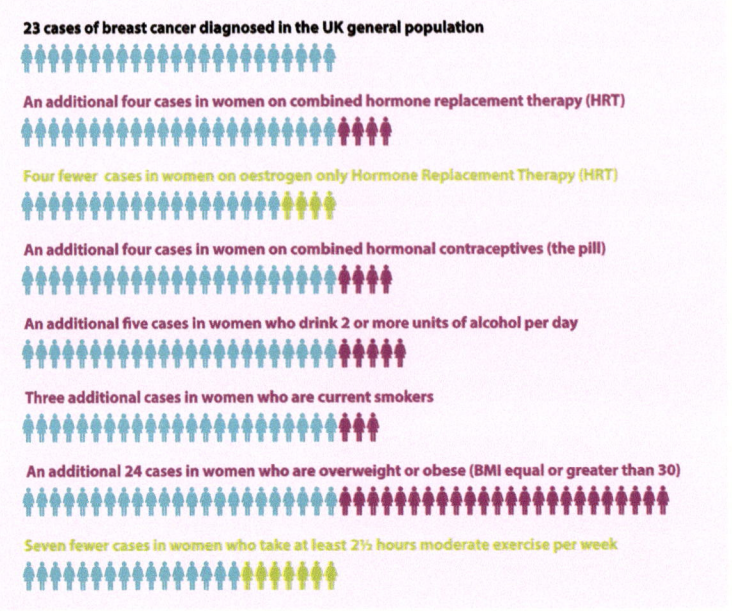

Figure 6.2 Difference in breast cancer incidence per 1,000 women aged 50–59. Approximate number of women developing breast cancer over the next five years. *Source*: BMS (2022). Reproduced with permission.

Cardiovascular risk (heart disease and stroke)
- No significant increase in the risk of CVD when started before 60 years of age and HRT may reduce the risk.
- Taking HRT tablets is associated with a very small increase in the risk of stroke (Hillard et al., 2021).

Prescribing and monitoring hormone replacement therapy

It is essential for any HCP who is going to specialise in the menopause to undertake training in this area. However, all HCPs can benefit by increasing their knowledge of the menopause in order to provide effective advice and care.

 Information on resources and CPD for healthcare professionals is provided on p. 83.

 A useful chart to aid in prescribing HRT has been produced by the BMS (Stephens et al., 2021).

The NICE clinical knowledge summary on HRT (NICE, 2022d) provides information on the following.

- Contraindications and cautions
- Route of administration
- Choice of hormone*
- Regimen
- Adverse effects.

*Important note: All people with a uterus taking unopposed oestrogen should take progestogen to prevent endometrial proliferation.

For those starting on HRT, follow-up in three months is advised. When providing care for women who are over the age of 50, there is an opportunity for HCPs to check whether they are using HRT and if so, to establish which regimen and whether appropriate monitoring is being undertaken. Annual review should include the following.

- Check for effectiveness of therapy and presence of side-effects, for example, breast tenderness, vaginal bleeding, nausea or headaches.
- Check blood pressure and weight.
- Encourage breast awareness and participation in screening.
- A review and discussion of an individual's risk–benefit ratio.
- If appropriate, consider switching from cyclical to continuous combined HRT.

A monthly withdrawal bleed is normal in women taking cyclical HRT and some irregular bleeding can be expected in the first three months of cyclical or continuous combined HRT. Any bleeding outside expected patterns will necessitate investigation to exclude abnormal pathology (Table 6.4). Investigations may include speculum and bimanual examination, TVUSS, endometrial biopsy/histology and hysteroscopy.

Table 6.4 Abnormal uterine bleeding in women taking HRT.

Regimen	Abnormal bleeding
Cyclical HRT users	If bleeding is persistently heavy or prolonged at the end or after the progestogen phase. If there is persistent breakthrough bleeding >6 months after starting HRT.
Continuous combined HRT users (unscheduled bleeding)	If persists >6 months of use or after 12 months of established amenorrhoea.

Sexual Health and Contraception

> Any unexplained vaginal bleeding in women who are not on HRT should also be investigated. The NICE Clinical Knowledge Summary: *Symptoms Suggestive of Gynaecological Cancers* (NICE, 2021a) recommends a suspected cancer pathway referral in the following presentations.
> - Postmenopausal bleeding in women age 55 years and over (unexplained vaginal bleeding more than 12 months after menstruation has stopped because of the menopause).
> - Postmenopausal bleeding in women age under 55 years (unexplained vaginal bleeding more than 12 months after menstruation has stopped because of the menopause).

See Chapter 5: Menstrual-Related Complications (pp. 55–69).

■ 'Alternatives' to Hormone Replacement Therapy

There are some women who cannot take HRT for medical reasons and others who do not wish to take it. Taking HRT is not the only treatment for the menopause and it should not be prescribed without considering other treatments and health-promoting lifestyle strategies. These health-enhancing activities will be familiar to HCPs as most are not 'alternative' but encouraged for everyone, including women who are prescribed HRT for menopause symptoms. They include recommending:

- a diet rich in calcium and healthy fats (such as avocado and nuts)
- reducing sugar and alcohol and limiting processed foods
- smoking and vaping cessation
- foods with a low glycaemic index (such as brown rice and oats)
- promoting gut health, which can have a positive influence on mood, emotions and well-being
- regular exercise to promote cardiovascular and bone health and reduce anxiety and stress
- promoting good sleep – avoiding caffeine a few hours before bedtime, no screens in the bedroom
- stress reduction therapies such as meditation, yoga, acupuncture and hypnotherapy.

Herbal preparations and supplements
- There has been little research in this area and products tend to vary in composition and potency. Herbal preparations should be clearly marked with the traditional herbal registration (THR) logo.
- Agnus castus, red clover and black cohosh may improve some symptoms such as mood swings, tension and anxiety.

Other prescribed medication

- Antidepressants can reduce hot flushes and night sweats in some women. Side-effects can include reduced libido and there is no evidence that taking antidepressants for low mood associated with menopause is beneficial.
- Gabapentin and pregabalin can be given for hot flushes with benefit for some women.
- Clonidine is sometimes given for hot flushes but is very seldom beneficial and side-effects can include lowering blood pressure and gastrointestinal disturbance.

■ Menopause Resources

For service users

- The 'Balance' website and app are freely available and offer a range of evidence-based resources about the menopause (Newson Health, 2023a).
- The website for 'Women's Health Concern' which is the patient arm of the BMS (Women's Health Concern, 2023).
- 'Menopause Matters' website. An independent website providing information on the menopause (Menopause Matters, 2023).

Resources and CPD for healthcare professionals

- The 'Balance' app and website (Newson Health, 2023a).
- 'Confidence in the Menopause' is a CPD accredited, remote education programme by Newson Health Research and Education It is aimed at any HCP who would like to formalise and accredit their learning and consulting skills around menopause care. It provides several menopause-related case studies, including videos using actors and HCPs (Newson Health, 2023b).
- 'The Newson Health Menopause Society' is a multidisciplinary team of HCPs and experts who are passionate about improving and understanding women's hormone health (Newson Health, 2023c).
- The course provided by the BMS – 'Principles and Practice of Menopause Care (PPMC)' programme – is recognised throughout the UK as the leading provider of certificated menopause and post-reproductive health education and training for HCPs (BMS, 2023).
- 'Essentials of Menopause Care' is a new course provided by the FSRH. It is aimed specifically at healthcare practitioners working in primary care settings; this course may act as a starting point for many while also providing a useful update for more experienced staff (FSRH, 2023c).
- *Management of the Menopause* by Hillard et al. (2021).
- 'Menopause – Guidance on management and prescribing HRT for GPs', produced by the Primary Care Women's Health Forum (Shaw, 2020).

CHAPTER **7**

Sexually Transmitted Infections

■ Introduction

Most methods of contraception do not protect patients from STIs. The impact of STIs remains greatest in young heterosexual people, 15–24 years of age; people from black and ethnic minority groups; and gay and bisexual men and other MSM (PHE, 2019). Reliable and correct use of condoms can significantly reduce the risk of STIs and it is important to promote the availability of condoms by local services, including through condom distribution schemes. Individuals who misuse alcohol/drugs, participate in sexual activity at a young age and who persistently have UPSI (sometimes referred to as 'condomless sex') with multiple partners are also at increased risk (NICE, 2022e). Regular testing for HIV and STIs is essential for good sexual health and patients should be encouraged to have an STI screen annually if they are having UPSI with new or casual partners (PHE, 2019).

 BASHH is an excellent resource for managing STIs (BASHH, 2022).

■ History Taking

- Does your patient have any symptoms of an STI? Consider STIs as a differential diagnosis (for example, to a UTI).
  - Are they well in themselves?
- Are they a sexual contact of someone with a recently confirmed STI?
- Ask for more detail about the sexual contact (gender, age, more than once, high-risk sexual activity, new partner).
- Do they use condoms?
- Have they previously been tested for an STI/HIV?
- Is EC indicated?
- Have they been generally unwell for a long period of time?

85

For additional information on sexual history taking, including suggested sequence of core questions and how to ask them, see Chapter 1: Communication (pp. 1–12).

Untreated STIs can lead to premature rupture of membranes in pregnancy.

Vaginal discharge can be a good indicator of certain pathophysiology. See pp. 15–16 in Chapter 2: Anatomy and Physiology – A Recap for physiology of normal vaginal discharge.

Table 7.1 identifies the features of vaginal discharge to be aware of and their related pathophysiology.

Table 7.1 Identifying pathophysiology in vaginal discharge.

Type of vaginal discharge	Possible association	Other symptoms
Milky or white with no odour	Physiological	None.
Thick white, may resemble cottage cheese	Vaginal yeast infection (Candida)	Vaginal itching, burning, soreness and/or pain. Can include dysuria and dyspareunia, vulval swelling or rash.
White, yellow or grey	Bacterial vaginosis (BV)	Malodour, often 'fishy'. Itching and swelling.
Yellow or green, frothy	Trichomoniasis vaginalis	Malodour.
An unusual vaginal discharge, may be watery and green or yellow	Gonorrhoea	Pelvic pain.
Brown or bloody	Irregular menstruation	Pelvic pain and/or vaginal bleeding. Irregular vaginal bleeding always warrants further investigation. See Menstrual-Related Complications chapters.

CHAPTER 7 • Sexually Transmitted Infections

A useful NHS resource for patients on vaginal discharge can be found online (NHS, 2021e). It contains information on what is normal and abnormal vaginal discharge and what to do and what not to do to manage discharge.

Examination

Depending on how the patient is in themselves, it may be appropriate to undertake vital observations. Conditional on the symptoms, it may be appropriate to undertake an examination of the external genitalia (always offer a chaperone) (for example, for genital herpes). It may also be appropriate to examine the abdomen (for example, for PID). Where appropriate, examine for lymphadenopathy and rashes and consider swabs and urinalysis.

For all STIs, the patient's partner(s) must also be treated to reduce the risk of onward transmission, and it is important that the patient is encouraged to have this discussion with associated contact/s. If the person is unwilling or unable to have this conversation, advise them that (with their consent) their details can be provided to their local sexual health service solely for the purposes of partner notification.

Online testing

Multiplex diagnostic assays are being used by online and private providers to test inappropriately for some organisms. Some providers offer treatment regimens which are inconsistent with national recommendations for first-line therapy. BASHH recommends that all STI service providers follow BASHH national clinical guidance for STI testing and offer first-line treatment to all patients with an STI where possible.

Types of Sexually Transmitted Infection

Chlamydia

Aetiology

Chlamydia is a bacterial infection and is one of the most common STIs in the UK. Two-thirds of chlamydia diagnoses are made in young people aged between 15 and 24, with an increase of 2% from 2018 (PHE, 2019). Anyone under 25 years of age who is sexually active should be screened for chlamydia on change of sexual partner or annually. An individual can contract chlamydia even if there is no penetration, orgasm or ejaculation. It can also be contracted

87

from infected semen or vaginal fluid getting into the eye and can be passed by a pregnant woman to her baby.

History and examination

A detailed history may be sufficient to obtain a diagnosis, taking symptoms into consideration, which can include dysuria, abnormal discharge (men and women), lower abdominal pain, post-coital or IMB in women, deep dyspareunia and pelvic pain in women, and pain or swelling of the testicles in men.

> Seventy percent of the time, chlamydia presents with no symptoms. If left undetected and untreated, complications such as PID and infertility can occur. It can also increase the risk of ectopic pregnancy. Be alert to the possibility of PID in women who are unwell with a history indicative of and symptoms consistent with chlamydia.

Diagnosis is confirmed with positive swabs in women (NAATs, nucleic acid amplification test) either that the patient has taken themselves or you as the clinician if trained to do so (vulvo-vaginal swab is normally the test of choice in most women). The swab needs to be inserted about 5 cm into the vagina and gently rotated for 10 seconds. In men, a first-catch urine is the specimen of choice.

> As the window period for chlamydia is up to two weeks, if the exposure was within the last two weeks, a test should be carried out at presentation and if negative, repeated two weeks after the exposure.

Management

Chlamydia is treated with antibiotics and your local antimicrobial prescribing guidelines. BASHH and NICE guidance should be followed if the prescription is undertaken in primary care, or referral to a sexual health clinic. Differences in treatment exist for those with allergies, and for patients who are pregnant or breastfeeding. Some key points for treatment and onwards care are listed below (NICE, 2021b).

- For pregnant women, management may be discussed with other HCPs involved in the woman's care (such as the woman's midwife and obstetrician), if the patient consents.
- If chlamydia is diagnosed in a child under 16 years, then discuss management with a primary care provider, sexual health specialist or paediatrician.
- The patient's current partner(s) must also be treated for chlamydia to reduce the risk of onward transmission.
- Advise patients not to have any sexual contact (including oral sex, genital contact, mutual masturbation or penetration, even if a condom is used) for the duration of treatment for both the patient and their partner(s), or seven days, whichever is longer.

CHAPTER 7 • Sexually Transmitted Infections

- Reinforce health education and the importance of condom use. Consider full STI screening if the patient consents to this; NAATs screen for both chlamydia and gonorrhoea.

Test of cure is not routinely recommended for uncomplicated genital chlamydia infection but is indicated in pregnancy, where poor compliance is suspected and where symptoms persist.

- Offer repeat testing to all people under the age of 25 years diagnosed with chlamydia 3–6 months after completion of treatment to check for reinfection.
- Consider offering repeat testing to people over the age of 25 years who are at high risk of reinfection.

The National Chlamydia Screening Programme (NCSP) is changing to focus on reducing reproductive harm of untreated infection in young women. Opportunistic screening should focus on women only. Men will not be proactively offered a test unless an indication has been identified, such as being a partner of someone with chlamydia or having symptoms (PHE, 2021).

If the patient is unwell with PID, refer them to genitourinary medicine/the ED.

Gonorrhoea

Aetiology

There was a 26% increase in gonorrhoea between 2017 and 2018, especially in young people. It is caused by a bacterium called *Neisseria gonorrhoeae* or *N. gonococcus*. Infection is transmitted vaginally or through oral sex and can occur in the urethra, cervix, rectum, throat and eyes with an incubation period of 1–4 days. The infection can also be passed from a pregnant woman to her baby. Without treatment, gonorrhoea can cause permanent blindness in a newborn baby (PHE, 2019).

History and examination

Symptoms present differently in men and women as outlined in Table 7.2.

- NAAT should be arranged for the presence of *N. gonorrhoeae* in line with local procedures and protocols.
- In women, a vulvo-vaginal swab (which may be self-taken) should be used. In men, a first-pass urine specimen should be used.
- Tests should be taken no earlier than three days after sexual contact with an infected person.
- Symptomatic patients or those who are contacts should have swabs for culture and sensitivities.

Table 7.2 Symptoms of gonorrhea in men and women.

Sex	Symptoms
Men	• Genital gonorrhoea infection is usually symptomatic in men. • Urethral infection causes mucopurulent or purulent urethral discharge in more than 80% of men, and dysuria in more than 50% of men within 2–5 days of exposure; usually there is no effect on frequency or urgency of urination. • Rectal infection is usually asymptomatic, but may cause anal discharge (12% of men), acute proctitis, peri-anal/anal pain or discomfort (7% of men), tenesmus or rectal bleeding. • Pharyngeal infection is asymptomatic in more than 90% of men, but may cause tonsillitis or pharyngitis. • Other symptoms may be caused by complications of gonorrhoea infection, including prostatitis, epididymitis and orchitis.
Women	• Urogenital gonorrhoea is asymptomatic in up to 50% of women. • Where present, symptoms usually develop within 10 days. • Increased or altered vaginal discharge (up to 50% of women). • Lower abdominal pain (up to 25% of women). • Dysuria (up to 12% of women); usually there is no effect on frequency of urination. • IMB or menorrhagia (rarely). • Dyspareunia if the infection spreads from the endocervix. • Pharyngeal infection is asymptomatic in 90% of women, but it may cause tonsillitis or pharyngitis.

Source: NICE (2022e).

Management

Gonorrhoea is rarely treated in primary care and the patient should be referred to a sexual health clinic for treatment, management and follow up. This is because gonorrhoea treatment is often not readily available and swabs for sensitivities need to be taken and followed up (NICE, 2020).

Genital herpes

Aetiology

Genital herpes is passed on through vaginal, anal and oral sex and is caused by the herpes simplex virus. It can range from being mild to very painful.

History and examination

Diagnosis is based on the presence of the following symptoms, in conjunction with a viral swab from the base of one of the lesions formed, which is sent for viral culture. Whilst the incubation period is 2–14 days, sometimes symptoms do not appear for years after first exposure (that is, not necessarily from a current/recent partner). Symptoms of genital herpes are as follows.

- Small blisters that burst to leave red, open sores around the genitals, anus, thighs or bottom.
- Lesions often develop 4–7 days after exposure to herpes simplex, but sometimes symptoms do not appear for years after first exposure (that is, not necessarily from a current/recent partner).
- Tingling, burning or itching around the genitals.
- Dysuria.
- Sometimes malaise or fever.
- Inguinal lymphadenopathy.
- Recurrent episodes usually occur in the same area and may be preceded by localised prodromal tingling and burning symptoms up to 48 hours before the appearance of lesions.

Management

Oral antivirals are the primary treatment for genital herpes simplex infection. Treatment should commence within five days of the start of the episode, or while new lesions are forming for people with a first clinical episode of genital herpes. If new lesions are still forming after 3–5 days, seek specialist advice.

Advise individuals about self-care measures, including taking adequate pain relief, washing the area with plain or salt water, applying Vaseline® or topical lidocaine, increase fluid intake to dilute the urine and avoid wearing tight clothing. Advise the patient to abstain from sex until the lesions have cleared.

If the infection is severe, the person is systemically unwell or complications are suspected (such as urinary retention), admit for treatment in secondary care (NICE, 2023).

Herpes simplex virus remains dormant. Some people have no recurrences. In line with BASHH guidance, suppression treatment can be offered to patients who have frequent occurrences (more than 6/year).

The Herpes Virus Association (2022) is a valuable resource for both HCPs and patients. It should be offered to all patients where herpes simplex virus is discussed, particularly the first episodes or those with recurrences.

It is vital to address the importance of interpersonal skills to minimise the stigma and address myths and misconceptions around the herpes simplex virus.

Transmission can occur when there are no symptoms (asymptomatic shedding), but the risk is higher when symptomatic.

Genital warts

Aetiology

Genital warts are usually asymptomatic, may be single or multiple and tend to occur in areas of high friction. The patient will present with local irritation and discomfort where warts occur and warts usually present as soft cauliflower-like growths of varying size.

History and examination

Diagnosis is made if there are one or more painless growths or lumps around the vulva, penis or anus. There may be itching or bleeding from the genitals or anus and a change in the normal flow of urine.

Management

- Refer people with anogenital warts to a sexual health specialist clinic if unable to manage in primary care.
- Treatment can be offered in primary care and is often topical (though these cannot be used in pregnancy, are not licensed in children and have a high likelihood of adverse effects).
- Sometimes treatment is not always indicated, as in about 30% of people, warts disappear spontaneously within four months (Leslie et al., 2023).
- Ablative methods (such as cryotherapy, excision and electrocautery) via a sexual health clinic.

Tracing of previous sexual partner(s) is not recommended for people with anogenital warts in the absence of other STIs (NHS, 2020b).

Trichomoniasis

Aetiology

Trichomoniasis is an STI caused by a tiny parasite called *Trichomonas vaginalis* (TV). It is the world's most common non-viral STI although relatively uncommon in the UK. Although symptoms of the infection vary, most people who have the parasite cannot tell they are infected.

History and examination

Symptoms of TV usually develop within a month of infection, but 50% of people will not develop any symptoms (though they can still pass the infection on to others) (NHS, 2021e). TV is not thought to be passed on through oral or anal sex. The symptoms of TV are similar to those of many other STIs and therefore

CHAPTER 7 · Sexually Transmitted Infections

Table 7.3 Symptoms of TV in women and men.

Sex	Symptoms
Women	• Abnormal vaginal discharge, typically, thin or frothy and yellow-green in colour. • Producing more discharge than normal, which may also have an unpleasant fishy smell (and can be misdiagnosed as BV). • Soreness, swelling and itching around the vagina. • Pain or discomfort when passing urine or having sexual intercourse.
Men	• Pain when urinating or during ejaculation. • Needing to urinate more frequently than usual. • Thin, white discharge from the penis. • Soreness, swelling and redness around the head of the penis or foreskin.

diagnosis can be difficult. There are differences in the symptoms of women and men which are presented in Table 7.3.

TV can be diagnosed from a swab taken from the vagina or penis on a wet-slide and microscopy. This test is often not available or practical in community settings. NAATs for TV are also not readily available and therefore TV is difficult to detect in primary care (40% sensitivity) – HCPs should therefore have a low threshold for referring to sexual health for more sensitive testing (NHS, 2018a).

Management

- Partner notification is essential to prevent reinfection. Current and recent partners should be tested and treated following a positive swab.
- TV is treated with antibiotics (refer to your local prescribing guidelines).

If a patient is infected with TV while they are pregnant, the infection may cause the baby to be born prematurely or have a low birth weight (NHS, 2018a).

Syphilis

Aetiology

Syphilis is a bacterial infection caused by the bacterium *Treponema pallidum* and is treated with a short course of antibiotics. There is a significant rise in rates of syphilis infection and clinicians should have a lower threshold for testing.

A patient can catch syphilis more than once. If left untreated, it can spread to the neurological system and cause serious long-term issues.

History and examination

Syphilis can present with a wide range of non-specific symptoms; in some people infection may be asymptomatic, therefore diagnosis can be delayed or missed. Common symptoms include the following.

- Small, (sometimes) painless sores or ulcers that typically appear on the penis, vagina or around the anus, but can occur in other places such as the mouth.
- A blotchy red rash that often affects the chest, palms of the hands or soles of the feet.
- Small skin growths (similar to genital warts) that may develop on the vulva in women or around the anus in both men and women.
- White patches in the mouth.
- Tiredness, headaches, joint pains, a fever, lymphadenopathy in the neck, groin or armpits, patchy alopecia, unilateral hearing loss and visual impairment.

Swabs from active lesions and serology confirm the diagnosis.

Management

Refer all people with syphilis to a specialist local sexual health service, as some tests are not available in primary care and the results are difficult to interpret (NICE, 2019c).

Hepatitis B

Aetiology

The hepatitis B virus is a major cause of serious, life-threatening liver disease, including liver cancer and cirrhosis. In 2017, the World Health Organization (WHO) estimated that around 250 million people worldwide were chronically infected with hepatitis B virus. Those at risk include people originally from high-risk countries, intravenous (IV) drug users, people who are HIV positive and people who have UPSI with multiple sexual partners (WHO, 2017). Hepatitis B vaccination is available for people at high risk of exposure to the condition.

History and examination

Symptoms can be generic, including tiredness, fever and general aches and pains, which normally begin 2–3 months after exposure. However, many patients can be asymptomatic. Hepatitis B should be considered in patients with a high risk of exposure and symptoms of:

- loss of appetite
- nausea and vomiting
- diarrhoea
- abdominal pain
- jaundice.

Diagnosis is confirmed with hepatitis B serology.

CHAPTER 7 • Sexually Transmitted Infections

Management

- Notify the health protection unit (HPU) promptly to facilitate appropriate surveillance and contact tracing.
- Admit any person with hepatitis B infection to hospital if they are severely unwell.
- Manage any pain, itching and nausea.
- Advise the patient to avoid drinking alcohol.
- Take steps to minimise transmission.
- Refer anyone who is found to be hepatitis B positive to a hepatologist, gastroenterologist or infectious disease specialist with specialism in hepatology (NICE, 2021c).

Human immunodeficiency virus

Aetiology

In the UK, about one in four of all new HIV infections occurs among young people aged 13–24 years and 73% of all infections are in men. Heterosexual people over 50 years of age are the fastest increasing group of new diagnoses (UK Health Security Agency, 2023). People can live well with HIV with early diagnosis and effective treatment, but without adequate treatment, AIDS-related illnesses can develop. HIV can be found in vaginal and anal fluids, breast milk, blood and semen; it cannot be transmitted through sweat, saliva or urine. Condomless anal and vaginal sex present the most common ways of transmitting the virus. HIV can also be transmitted through shared needles and between mother and child during pregnancy, birth or breastfeeding. Individuals most at risk include IV drug users, MSM and those with a partner from a high-risk country (National AIDs Trust, 2021).

Please refer to the HIV Lens website (HIV Lens, 2023) to assist you in establishing if you should be doing routine/opportunistic HIV screening, based on local prevalence data.

See pp. 7–8 in Chapter 1: Communication for examples of how to ask questions when taking a sexual history, particularly Box 1.5 Key questions when assessing the risk of BBVs.

Adult HIV Testing Guidelines (BHIVA, 2020).

History and examination

HIV must be considered in patients from the high-risk groups who have unexplained symptoms that are unusually prolonged, severe or recurrent. Consider HIV in patients with lymphadenopathy, weight loss and persistent pyrexia of unknown origin. Increasingly, virologists will advise testing for

HIV on requests for cytomegalovirus (CMV), Epstein-Barr virus (EBV), 'glandular fever' and viral hepatitis. Primary HIV infection presents with fever, sore throat, maculopapular rash, malaise, lethargy, arthralgia, myalgia, lymphadenopathy and oral, genital or peri-anal ulcers and less commonly with headache, meningitis, cranial nerve palsies, diarrhoea and weight loss.

Conditions associated with longstanding HIV infection can be subtle and people may remain well for some time before developing another condition.

HIV testing should be considered in the following situations: sexual risk, physical symptoms, a partner who tested HIV positive, a routine STI investigation, antenatal screening, an initial or change in sexual partner, discontinuation or no condom use, patient concern, sexual assault, blood donation and occupational exposure. British HIV Association (BHIVA) guidelines suggest that HCPs need to integrate HIV testing more readily into a routine work-up for patients as this helps to normalise HIV testing (BHIVA, 2020).

Diagnosis is confirmed with HIV serology.

The significance of the window period as a repeat test may be necessary. The window period is the time between becoming infected and antibodies appearing; HIV antibodies usually appear 4–6 weeks after infection but can take up to 12 weeks. Therefore, you may need to repeat the blood test.

Management

Management of the patient depends on whether this is a new diagnosis of HIV or management of PEP to reduce the chance of developing HIV infection.

A patient with a new diagnosis will need to be referred urgently to a specialist HIV clinic, to be seen preferably within 48 hours and at the latest within two weeks of testing positive.

Arrange admission for urgent specialist assessment if there is concern about the possibility of a serious HIV-related condition such as *Pneumocystis* pneumonia or the patient is unwell.

Treatment

Antiretroviral (ARV) therapy is prescribed to patients with a diagnosis of HIV. It helps to keep the viral load low. It can make the load so low that it is undetectable by a test. Undetectable equals untransmittable ('U=U'). A person living with HIV, who has an undetectable viral load, cannot pass HIV on to their sexual partners. This can:

- reduce HIV-related stigma
- improve mental/emotional health for people living with HIV
- reduce barriers to testing
- reduce time between infection and diagnosis
- prevent new infections.

Whilst initiation and management of ARV therapy are largely carried out by specialist HIV services, the HIV Drug Interactions website provided by the University of Liverpool offers useful guidance on drug interactions (University of Liverpool, 2022).

ARV should be:

- taken as soon as diagnosed
- taken every day.

It helps to:

- suppress viral replication
- enable immune recovery
- reduce morbidity and mortality
- stop transmission.

Post-exposure prophylaxis

PEP is a course of anti-HIV medication. It may stop a person from developing HIV if they have been exposed to the virus, but it does not always work. Direct the patient immediately to a sexual health clinic or an ED for consideration of PEP following sexual exposure.

The patient must start the treatment as soon as possible after they have been exposed to HIV, ideally within a few hours. The medicines must be taken every day for 28 days (four weeks). PEP is unlikely to work if it is started after three days (72 hours) and it will not usually be prescribed after this time. It is best to start taking PEP within one day (24 hours) of being exposed to HIV.

Pre-exposure prophylaxis

Pre-exposure prophylaxis (PrEP) is a medicine taken by individuals who are at risk of HIV infection. When PrEP is taken as prescribed, it is highly effective. The regimens for PrEP are either daily or event based – this is determined by patient preference and risk. BHIVA and BASHH provide evidence-based guidance on best clinical practice in the provision, monitoring and support of PrEP for the prevention of HIV acquisition (BHIVA/BASHH, 2018). All patients are offered a prescription, full STI screening including HIV testing and 3–12-monthly renal function check. Research suggests that PrEP is safe, but it is common for patients to suffer side-effects such as diarrhoea, nausea, headache, fatigue and abdominal pain. PrEP is approved for use by anyone without

HIV who weighs at least 35 kg and who is at risk of getting HIV from sex or injection drug use.

PrEP is:

- now fully available on the NHS – currently managed by and only available from specialist sexual health services
- the single most effective measure for preventing HIV – up to 100% effective at preventing HIV acquisition.

A patient may be indicated to have PrEP if any of the factors from Box 7.1 apply.

Health promotion

People with HIV attending primary care may require:

- advice about sources of information and support
- information on health promotion, screening and immunisation
- information on sexual and reproductive health
- management of mental health issues
- management of HIV-related problems
- support for end-stage advanced HIV disease.

Box 7.1 Indications for PrEP

Recommend PrEP

(i) HIV-negative MSM and trans women who report condomless anal sex in the previous six months and ongoing condomless anal sex.
(ii) HIV-negative individuals having UPSI with partners who are HIV positive, unless the partner has been on ARV therapy for at least six months and their plasma viral load is <200 copies/ml.

Consider PrEP on a case-by-case basis

PrEP may be offered on a case-by-case basis to HIV-negative individuals considered at increased risk of HIV acquisition through a combination of factors that may include the following.

Population-level indicators

- Heterosexual black African men and women.
- Recent migrants to the UK.
- Transgender women.
- People who inject drugs.
- People who report sex work or transactional sex.

Clinical indicators

- Rectal bacterial STI in the previous year.
- Bacterial STI or hepatitis C virus (HCV) in the previous year.
- Post-exposure prophylaxis following sexual exposure (PEPSE) in the previous year, particularly where repeated courses have been used.

Box 7.1 *(Continued)*

Sexual behaviour/sexual network indicators

- High-risk sexual behaviour: reporting UPSI with partners of unknown HIV status, and particularly where this is condomless anal sex or with multiple partners.
- UPSI with partners from a population group or country with high HIV prevalence.
- UPSI with sexual partners who may fit the criteria of 'high risk of HIV'.
- Engages in chemsex or group sex.
- Reports anticipated future high-risk sexual behaviour.
- Condomless vaginal sex should only be considered high risk where other contextual factors or vulnerabilities are present.

Drug use

- Sharing injecting equipment.
- Injecting in an unsafe setting.
- No access to needle and syringe programmes or opioid substitution therapy.

Sexual health autonomy

Other factors that may affect sexual health autonomy:

- Inability to negotiate and/or use condoms (or employ other HIV prevention methods) with sexual partners.
- Coercive and/or violent power dynamics in relationships (for example, intimate partner/domestic violence).
- Precarious housing or homelessness, and/or other factors that may affect material circumstances.
- Risk of sexual exploitation and trafficking.

Source: Brady et al. (2019).

To assist with mental health support or if a patient is suffering from a long-term condition, consider engagement with a local health and well-being group or input from a social prescriber or link worker (NICE, 2021d). The Terrence Higgins Trust is a useful resource for further support (Terrence Higgins Trust, 2023).

■ Common Vaginal Infections

Bacterial vaginosis

Aetiology

BV is common and is caused by a change in the natural balance of bacteria in the vagina; what causes this to happen is not fully known.

Advise the patient that BV is not an STI, as this often leads to apprehension and confusion and is not always common knowledge (although it can be triggered by sexual intercourse).

History and examination

Approximately 50% of women with BV are asymptomatic (Coudray and Madhivanan, 2019), but when symptoms do exist, BV often presents as a malodourous, thin, grey/white homogeneous discharge that is not associated with itching or soreness.

Management

Management information has been based on NICE (2018c).

- If empirical treatment is not considered appropriate or the diagnosis is uncertain, examine the woman and arrange investigations.
- Take a vaginal swab to exclude other causes of symptoms from all women of reproductive age with vaginal discharge.
- If the woman is asymptomatic, treatment is not usually required, unless she is undergoing an abortion.
- If the woman is symptomatic, advise that, where possible, she should reduce exposure to contributing factors, such as excessive vaginal washing and the use of antiseptics, products labelled for 'genital hygiene', bubble baths, soap or shampoos.
- Prescribe oral metronidazole 400 mg twice a day for 5–7 days.
- If adherence to treatment is an issue, a single oral dose of 2 grams may be used, if appropriate.
- If the woman prefers topical treatment or cannot tolerate oral metronidazole then you can prescribe intravaginal metronidazole gel 0.75% once a day for five days (off-label for women aged younger than 18 years) or intravaginal clindamycin cream 2% once a day for seven days.

 High-dose regimens (single oral dose of 2 grams) are not recommended during pregnancy.

Candida

Aetiology

Candida, commonly referred to as 'thrush', is a very frequent presentation in primary care for both men and women. Like BV, it is not classified as an STI.

History and examination

Symptoms in women include:

- white vaginal discharge (often like cottage cheese), which does not usually smell
- itching and irritation around the vagina
- soreness and stinging during sex or when passing urine.

CHAPTER 7 · Sexually Transmitted Infections

A vaginal examination is not normally required but if symptoms are recurrent and severe, a genital examination could be offered.

Symptoms in men include:

- irritation, burning and redness around the head of the penis and under the foreskin
- a white discharge (like cottage cheese)
- an unpleasant smell
- difficulty pulling back the foreskin.

Management

- Thrush can be managed by local pharmacies so encourage this with your patient.
- Advise self-management measures, such as using simple emollient and avoiding overwashing, the use of scented washing products and soap and wearing tight-fitting clothes.
- Antifungal treatment such as cream, pessary or an oral tablet can be used depending on the symptoms and patient preference.

For patients presenting with recurrent thrush, always screen for diabetes.

Always assess the patient's risk of STIs when they present with potential thrush or BV.

CASE STUDY

Presenting complaint

A 28-year-old male presents to you with dysuria.

History

History of presenting complaint

- He is well in himself with no fever, no abdominal pain, no loin pain and no testicular pain.
- He tells you there is no discharge, itching, swelling, sores, warts or erythema to his penis.
- He has never had a UTI before.
- Previous STI screen (chlamydia and gonorrhoea) about two years ago was negative.
- He has had UPSI with multiple partners since he was 18 years old.
- He once paid to have sex with a man when he was 21.
- He has recently had UPSI with two new partners (both women) in the last month.

- He tells you that one of the recent partners thought that she might have chlamydia.

Past medical/family/drug history
- None, normally fit and well, no regular medicines.

Social history
- Smoker: 20 per day.
- Works as a scaffolder.

Examination
- His urine shows no nitrites, no leucocytes, no blood, no protein and no glucose on dipping. It appears clear.
- His observations are all within healthy ranges.

Preferred diagnosis
- Chlamydia.

Differential diagnoses
- UTI
- Non-specific urethritis
- TV
- Gonorrhoea.

Management
- You strongly suspect an STI (chlamydia) and as a contact, test and treat him for chlamydia.
- You arrange a first-catch urine NAAT for chlamydia and gonorrhoea to confirm diagnosis.
- You prescribe doxycycline 100 mg twice daily for seven days (first-line treatment) as there are no contraindications and it is within your scope of practice to prescribe.
- His current partner(s) must also be treated for chlamydia to reduce the risk of reinfection and onward transmission. You discuss partner notification with him; he is in contact with both recent sexual partners and agrees to notify them – this will include advising them to get tested and treated as a contact of chlamydia.
- You explain that sexual, genital contact (including oral sex, mutual masturbation even with a condom) should be avoided until he and his partner(s) have completed treatment (or waited seven days after treatment with azithromycin).
- You give him written advice (for example, BASHH 'A Guide to Chlamydia') and discuss safer sex.
- Due to his high-risk sexual activity, he agrees to further screening (gonorrhoea, HIV, hepatitis B and C and syphilis).
- He will call for his results to confirm the chlamydia diagnosis and check the results of other tests.

CHAPTER 8

Safeguarding

Emma Painter

■ Introduction

Safeguarding is everyone's responsibility (HM Government, 2018). The British Association for Sexual Health and HIV (Ashby et al., 2021) tells us that good-quality sexual health consultations are about building a good relationship with patients. We are often already asking intimate questions so by ensuring that safeguarding is on our radar, we can take each important opportunity to ensure topics such as domestic or sexual violence, honour-based violence, feeling safe in your home and child sexual exploitation are thought about.

Safeguarding in sexual health can often involve managing uncertainty – both ours and the patient's. We can feel there is a conflict between sustaining the fragile rapport we have built with our patient and carrying out our safeguarding responsibilities. Here are some examples of common anxieties that may be barriers to safeguarding.

- Ignoring the feeling that something is not OK because you do not have time to ask more questions.
- Being concerned that you will not know what to do if a patient tells you something that you need to act on.
- Not acting because you do not know where to seek support.

In any consultation, you should be alert to potential signs of abuse. In adults, there are ten categories of abuse (Care Act 2014) (Figure 8.1).

In this chapter, we will explore abuse and safeguarding concerns within the context of sexual health. Once the legislation has been laid out and understood, this will be explored through several key safeguarding scenarios in sexual health.

Sexual Health and Contraception

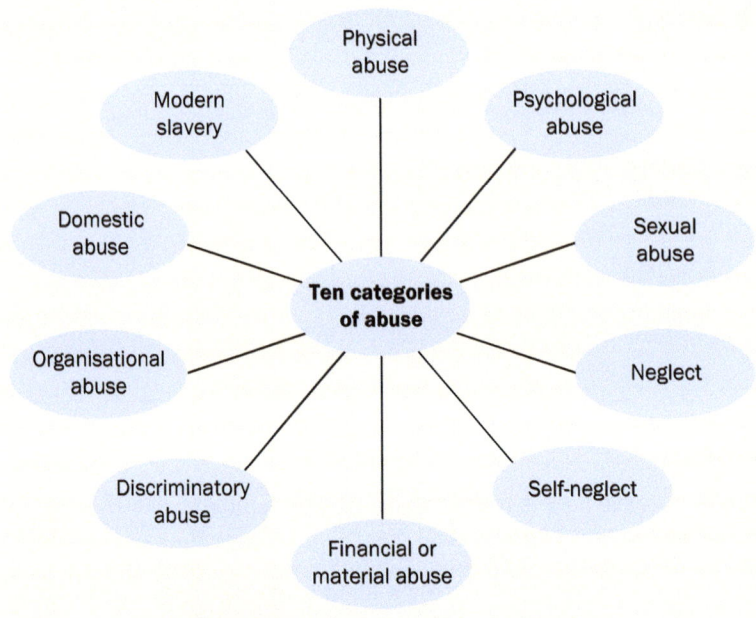

Figure 8.1 Ten categories of abuse.

Reflective activity

Whilst reading this chapter, it is likely that you will reflect on consultations or interactions that you have had with patients; you might find it useful to briefly note these down as an activity to enhance your learning. You can use these notes as the basis for finding out about local support services and perhaps to share your questions, and learning, with colleagues.

■ Regional Variability in Support Services

Whilst safeguarding guidance is national, referral pathways, advice and support services will vary regionally. A comprehensive understanding of safeguarding issues and resources will help you to feel confident when you see patients who trigger your professional curiosity concerning potential safeguarding issues.

■ Six Principles of Safeguarding Work

There are six principles which underpin all safeguarding work (Care Act 2014). We have a duty of care to patients, and a professional responsibility to follow these principles during our patient interactions. Table 8.1 puts these principles into a patient context.

Table 8.1 Six principles of safeguarding work.

Principle	Definition	The patient's perspective
Empowerment	People being supported and encouraged to make their own decisions and give informed consent.	'I am asked what I want as the outcomes from the safeguarding process and these directly inform what happens.'
Prevention	It is better to take action before harm occurs.	'I receive clear and simple information about what abuse is, how to recognise the signs and what I can do to seek help.'
Proportionality	The least intrusive response appropriate to the risk presented.	'I am sure that the professionals will work in my interest, as I see them and they will only get involved as much as needed.'
Protection	Support and representation for those in greatest need.	'I get help and support to report abuse and neglect. I get help so that I am able to take part in the safeguarding process to the extent to which I want.'
Partnership	Local solutions through services working with their communities. Communities have a part to play in preventing, detecting and reporting neglect and abuse.	'I know that staff treat any personal and sensitive information in confidence, only sharing what is helpful and necessary. I am confident that professionals will work together and with me to get the best result for me.'
Accountability	Accountability and transparency in delivering safeguarding.	'I understand the role of everyone involved in my life and so do they.'

■ Key Concepts in Safeguarding Relevant to Sexual Health

Sexual Offences Act 2003

Concerning causing a person to engage in sexual activity without consent, section 4.1 of the Sexual Offences Act 2003 states:

(1) A person (A) commits an offence if –
  (a) [They] intentionally cause another person (B) to engage in an activity,
  (b) the activity is sexual,
  (c) B does not consent to engaging in the activity, and
  (d) A does not reasonably believe that B consents.

Children under 13 are not legally able to consent to any form of sexual activity. A person aged 18 or over is committing an offence if they are having sex, or sexual contact, or inciting that child to have sex, sexual contact, or watch a sexual act:

- *with a child who is under 16 years of age, and who they do not reasonably believe to be 16 years old or over*

OR

- *if the child is under 13 years of age.*

When considering and discussing safeguarding cases, it can be useful to always call patients who are under 18 years of age 'children'. Similarly, it can be helpful to reverse the gender of your patient when thinking about your concerns and see if that alters how you are thinking about the case. For example, if you are working with a 15-year-old boy and you are unsure if you need to act on your concerns, consider what you would do if it was a 15-year-old girl. Both of these tips can help put your concerns in perspective, and also describe and escalate things appropriately. It can also be a good way to challenge and escalate things with social care if necessary.

Mental Capacity Act 2005

The Mental Capacity Act 2005 provides a framework for working with people aged 16 years and over when considering if they have the ability to consent to or refuse treatment. There are five key principles contained within the Act, which all HCPs must abide by (Table 8.2).

Table 8.2 Five key principles of the Mental Capacity Act 2005.

Principle	Description
1. Presumption of capacity	Assume a person has the capacity to make a decision themselves, unless it is proven otherwise.
2. Individuals being supported to make their own decisions	Wherever possible, help people to make their own decisions.
3. Unwise decisions	Do not treat a person as lacking the capacity to make a decision just because they make an unwise decision.
4. Best interests	If you make a decision for someone who does not have capacity, it must be in their best interests.
5. Least restrictive option	Treatment and care provided to someone who lacks capacity should be the least restrictive of their basic rights and freedoms.

Adults with Incapacity (Scotland) Act 2000

The Adults with Incapacity (Scotland) Act 2000 provides a similar framework for working with people aged 16 years and over in Scotland, when considering if they have the ability to consent to or refuse treatment. There are five key principles contained within the Act, which all HCPs must abide by (Table 8.3).

Table 8.3 Five key principles of the Adults with Incapacity (Scotland) Act 2000.

Principle	Description
1. Benefit	Any action or decisions taken must benefit the adult and only be taken when that benefit cannot reasonably be achieved without it.
2. Least restrictive option	Any action or decision taken should be the minimum necessary to achieve the purpose. It should be the option that restricts the person's freedom as little as possible.
3. Take account of the wishes of the adult	In deciding if an action or decision is to be made, and what that should be, account shall be taken of the present and past wishes and feelings of the adult as far as they can be ascertained. The adult should be offered appropriate assistance to communicate their views.
4. Consultation with relevant others	In deciding if an action or decision is to be made, and what that should be, account shall be taken of the views of the nearest relative and the primary carer of the adult, the adult's named person, any guardian or attorney with powers relating to the proposed intervention, and any person whom the Sheriff has directed should be consulted, in so far as it is reasonable and practicable to do so.
5. Encouraging the adult	Any guardian, attorney, or manager of an establishment exercising functions under the Act shall in so far as it is reasonable and practicable to do so, encourage the adult to exercise whatever skills they have concerning property, financial affairs or personal welfare as the case may be and to develop new such skills.

Mental Capacity Act (Northern Ireland) 2016

The Mental Capacity Act (Northern Ireland) 2016 provides statutory principles for working with people aged 16 years and over in Northern Ireland, when considering if they have the ability to consent to or refuse treatment. There are five statutory principles contained within the Act, which all HCPs must abide by (Table 8.4).

Table 8.4 Five statutory principles of the Mental Capacity Act (Northern Ireland) 2016.

Principle	Description
1. No one should be treated as lacking capacity unless it is proven they do	A person who is thinking about carrying out a deprivation of liberty must not misinterpret the first Principle as requiring them to presume or assume that the person has capacity or that the person lacks capacity. The Principle places the onus on a person intending to carry out the DoL to have properly established a person's capacity. However, the starting point when establishing capacity should be that the person has capacity.
2. No assumptions can be made	The Principle forbids any assumptions based merely on any condition that the person has or any other characteristics of the person. Such a condition or characteristic may be a disability, age, appearance, physical or mental illness or anything else. Just because a person presents symptoms of a condition that often, or sometimes, can suggest a person lacks capacity cannot be used as the reasoning for establishing or concluding that the person lacks capacity.
3. Help and support must be provided	This Principle requires that anyone who is considering whether a person lacks capacity must consider and provide all practicable help and support to allow the person to make their own decision. No determination of lack of capacity can be made until all practicable help and support has been provided. This helps individuals to play as big a role as possible in the decision making process to retain as much autonomy as possible.
4. No assumptions can be made because of unwise decisions	All persons have their own wishes, feelings, beliefs and values. No one should be assumed to lack capacity just because they make a decision that to others may appear unwise. This applies even if family members, friends, health and social care staff or others are unhappy with the decision. Unwise decisions are even allowed if the decision is one that could have negative effects on the person making the decision.

CHAPTER 8 • Safeguarding

Table 8.4 (Continued)

Principle	Description
5. All acts and decisions must be made in the person's best interests	The fifth Principle requires any act done or decision made on behalf of a person who is 16 or over and lacks capacity, to be in that person's best interests. The person determining best interests is required, so far as is practicable, to encourage and help the person to participate as fully as possible in the decision making process. **Special regard must be given to the person's values and beliefs, and past and present wishes and feelings.** The person determining best interests must also consult with others and take into account their views as to what would be in the best interests of the person who lacks capacity. The person determining best interests must also have regard to any less restrictive alternatives to the proposed deprivation of liberty.

Gillick Competence and Fraser Guidelines

Gillick Competence and Fraser Guidelines help HCPs work with patients who are children. They are the result of legal action brought in the 1980s by a parent, Mrs Gillick, and the resulting guidelines written by Lord Fraser (Griffith, 2016). The Children Act 2004 defines a child as anyone who has not yet reached their 18th birthday.

What is Gillick Competence?

Gillick Competence refers to the assessment that should be made in relation to whether a child under the age of 16 has the understanding to consent to treatment without parental or guardian consent. This is relevant in England, Wales and Northern Ireland.

What are Fraser Guidelines?

Fraser Guidelines are specific to contraception. They are the result of Lord Fraser's involvement with the Gillick case. He commented on the responsibility of doctors to ensure adequate capacity of children specifically receiving contraceptive advice and prescriptions. Fraser Guidelines apply specifically to advice and treatment on contraception, sexual health, STIs and abortions.

Clinicians using the Fraser Guidelines should be satisfied that:
- the young person cannot be persuaded to inform their parents or carers they are seeking this advice or treatment and will not allow you to do this either

109

- the young person understands the advice given
- the young person's physical or mental health, or both, are likely to suffer unless they receive the advice or treatment
- it is in the young person's best interests to receive the advice, treatment or both without their parents' or carers' consent
- the young person is very likely to continue having sex with or without treatment.

The National Society for the Prevention of Cruelty to Children (NSPCC, 2022) reminds us that when using Fraser Guidelines, it is important to be mindful:

- of the possibility that a child is being sexually exploited or groomed
- that sexual activity with a child under 13 years of age is statutory rape, and should always result in a child protection referral (regardless of the age of the partner)
- that a child presenting with repeated STIs, abortions or pregnancy may indicate sexual abuse or exploitation.

> For further information on Gillick Competence and Fraser Guidelines see NSPCC Learning's (2022) *Gillick Competency and Fraser Guidelines* and the CQC's (2022) *GP Myth Buster 8: Gillick Competency and Fraser Guidelines*.

Confidentiality

The Nursing and Midwifery Council (NMC, 2023) and the Health and Care Professions Council (HCPC, 2016) both outline the importance of confidentiality in their standards. Some key points are as follows.

- Information is confidential to an organisation, not an individual. Never tell a patient that you can keep information confidential regardless of what it is.
- You do not need to gain consent to seek safeguarding advice or support from within your organisation.
- General Data Protection Regulations (GDPR) and/or information governance cannot be used as an excuse for not sharing relevant, important and proportionate safeguarding information.
- It is good practice to advise a patient, and gain consent, before sharing information. It is best to do this at the time the disclosure is made. Use simple language, being clear about who you are going to tell and what you think might happen, for example: 'I will need to share this information with social care. I am doing this to ensure that you and your family have all the support that you need. I will let social care know your feelings about this referral. Social care may get in contact to ask for more information. As part of sharing information with social care I will also let your health visitor/school nurse/school/mental health worker/support worker know'.
- You can share information HCP to HCP without consent. However, if you want the HCP you are sharing information with to take action, they may

not be able to do this without the patient knowing that information has been shared.

Think Family

'Think Family' recognises the importance of considering the whole family when working with patients. In practice, this means considering the following points.

- If working with an adult, assessing if their presenting problem may have an impact on any children or adults they are caring for. For example, the impact of domestic abuse between parents or guardians, or who is caring for a child or vulnerable adult whilst your patient is attending appointments.
- When working with a child, considering if they have any caring responsibilities, for example, are they a young carer?
- Trying to ensure that any support offered strengthens families.

This concept should not prevent HCPs from considering the individualised support that the patient in front of them requires.

For further information on Think Family, please see Social Care Institute for Excellence's (SCIE, 2011) *Think Child, Think Parent, Think Family: A guide to parental mental health and child welfare.*

■ Key Safeguarding Scenarios Related to Sexual Health

Sexual violence

This is any sexual act or activity (including online) which takes place without consent. It may include pressure, manipulation, bullying, intimidation, threats, deception and/or force (Rape Crisis, 2023).

Things to consider

- The majority of sexual violence takes place within relationships.
- Some patients may not consider what has happened or is happening to them to be sexual violence.
- 'Think Family' where children or vulnerable adults are present at the time of the sexual violence.
- Patients who are female, trans, in same-sex relationships or have physical or learning disabilities are considered at higher risk.
- If a child has been sexually assaulted or abused then this will need to be reported, either via social care or to the police, as a crime against a child has taken place.
- If an adult without capacity has been sexually assaulted or abused, then again this will need to be reported, either via social care or to the police.

Sexual Health and Contraception

- An adult with capacity can decide whether they wish to report a crime to the police.
  - Unless there is 'public interest', social care do not need to be advised.
  - Examples of public interest would include if the sexual assault or abuse was carried out by:
    - a trusted member of the local community, such as a religious leader
    - a person who holds a position of responsibility, such as an HCP, police officer, magistrate
    - someone who works with children, for instance a teacher or youth group leader.
  - In this case, the Local Authority Designated Officer (also known as the LADO) will need to be involved.
  - Depending on the process in your area, you, your safeguarding lead or social care will need to make this referral.

Professional obligations

- Believe what the patient tells you. You do not need to investigate – that is the role of the police.
- Attend to any physical injuries.
- Are there children or vulnerable adults in the home or present when the sexual violence is taking place? If so, this would require an automatic referral to social services.
- To make a follow-up plan with your patient, consider EC, PEP for HIV, PEP for hepatitis B and C, screening for STIs; a follow-up pregnancy test.
- Ensure the patient will be safe. Make a safety plan.
- Consider who you are sharing information with and why, and document your rationale.
- Stay up to date with child protection and adult safeguarding essential training.
- Make accurate, contemporaneous notes.

 Safety Planning (Women's Aid, 2022).

Support for the patient

- Find out who provides your local IDSVA services.

 For an excellent overview of the support available to patients, see Rape Crisis (2023) *Get Help*.

- Find out what services are available in your local area. This may include, but is not limited to your local SARC, counselling services (there may be specific services for girls and women, men and boys, trans and non-binary patients), your local sexual health service, police officers who specialise in sexual violence.
- If there are children in the home, consider sharing information with the school or school nurse and information on any other psychological support services available.

Domestic violence and abuse

This is defined by the Home Office (2012) as:

> 'any incident or pattern of incidents of controlling, coercive or threatening behaviour, violence or abuse between those aged 16 or over who are or have been intimate partners or family members regardless of gender or sexuality. This can encompass, but is not limited to, the following types of abuse: psychological, physical, sexual, financial, emotional'.

Things to consider

- 'Think Family'.
- The importance of safety planning.
- Victims of domestic abuse may need to be specifically asked a number of times before making a disclosure.
- Domestic abuse can affect all ages, genders, sexualities, religions, ethnicities and socioeconomic backgrounds.
- Patients who are female, trans, in same-sex relationships, or have physical or learning disabilities are considered at higher risk.
- Signs of domestic abuse may include being socially isolated, bruising and/or injuries, having no financial control, lack of freedom of movement and having communications or social media monitored.

Professional obligations

- Attend to any physical injuries.
- Are there children or vulnerable adults in the home or present when the violence or abuse is taking place? If so, this would require an automatic referral to social services.
- If there are no children or vulnerable adults in the home then your patient has a choice as to what happens next, unless you assess there is an imminent risk of major or catastrophic harm. In this case, you will need to refer to your local guidance, which may include referral to a Multi-Agency Risk Assessment Conference (MARAC) or the police.
- Ensure you have made appropriate referrals and consider psychological support.
- Ensure you have discussed a safety plan with the patient.
- Consider why and with whom you are sharing information.
- Stay up to date with child protection and adult safeguarding essential training.
- Make accurate, contemporaneous notes.

Support for the patient

> For up-to-date support services, see Home Office (2018) *Domestic Abuse: How to Get Help*. This has information about services in the different countries of the UK.

- Consider 'Clare's Law', also known as the Domestic Violence Disclosure Scheme, where you as an HCP, or any individual, can ask the police if a partner has a history of perpetrating domestic abuse.
- Find out who provides your local IDSVA services.
- If there are children in the home, consider sharing information with the school or school nurse and any psychological support for them.

Female genital mutilation

Female genital mutilation comprises all procedures involving partial or total removal of the external female genitalia or other injury to the female genital organs for non-medical reasons (WHO, 2022).

Things to consider

Table 8.5 describes and portrays the four different types of FGM as classified by the WHO.

Professional obligations

If a disclosure of FGM is made or FGM is noted during a physical examination then follow the procedure listed below.

- Assess any physical or psychological needs your patient may have.
- Assess any risk to female relatives, such as sisters, daughters or nieces.
- Carry out your mandatory recording duty.
  - The type of FGM that has taken place.
  - Age when FGM took place.
  - Family history of FGM.
  - If the patient has at-risk female relatives.
  - The patient has been advised that FGM is illegal.
- Provide the patient with written information, in their first language, if possible.
- If you believe there is any risk to a child then you must make an urgent safeguarding referral. If you believe there is an imminent risk then you may need to call the police. Always discuss this type of action with a senior colleague or your safeguarding lead.

If you need to make a safeguarding referral, tell the patient if it is safe to do so.

Support for the patient

For support services, please see NHS (2022c) *Female Genital Mutilation (FGM)* and NSPCC (2023a) *Female Genital Mutilation (FGM)*.

 The Department of Health document *Female Genital Mutilation Risk and Safeguarding: Guidance for professionals* (Department of Health, 2016) is a useful resource.

CHAPTER 8 • Safeguarding

Table 8.5 Types of FGM.

Type of FGM	Description	Diagram
Type I Clitoridectomy	Partial or total removal of the clitoris and/or prepuce (the clitoral hood or fold of skin surrounding the clitoris).	
Type II Excision	Partial or total removal of the clitoris and the inner labia, with or without excision of the outer labia.	
Type III Infibulation	Narrowing of the vaginal opening by creating a covering seal. The seal is formed by cutting and repositioning the inner or outer labia, with or without removal of the clitoris.	
Type IV Other	All other harmful procedures to the female genitalia for non-medical purposes, for example pricking, piercing, incising, scraping and cauterising (burning) the genital area.	Burning / Pricking / Piercing

Child sexual exploitation

Child sexual exploitation (CSE) is a type of sexual abuse, where a child is given things, for example gifts, money, affection, in exchange for performing sexual acts (NSPCC, 2023b).

Things to consider

A perpetrator of CSE can be any age or gender. Signs of CSE may include STIs; sexual assault, repeated pregnancy risks, lack of contraception or repeated abortions, medically unexplained symptoms, physical assaults, missing school, becoming distanced from family and friends, changes in behaviour, new or increased alcohol or drug use, an increase in spending money or unexplained gifts.

Some key terms to consider in this context are listed below.

- Grooming: a child is tricked into believing they are in a true consensual relationship (NSPCC, 2023b).
- Trafficking: if two of the following have taken place for the purposes of exploitation: recruitment, transportation, harbouring (Children's Society, 2021).

Professional obligations

- Always consider the safety of the child first.
- Ask about other children at risk, for example siblings or friends.
- Urgently liaise with a senior colleague or your local safeguarding lead.
- If there is immediate risk to that child then strongly consider making contact with the police.
- You must make a social care referral.
- Know what your local processes are, both within your place of work and the local area.
- Consider who you are sharing information with and why.
- Stay up to date with child protection essential training (as stipulated in your practice's safeguarding policy).
- Make accurate, contemporaneous notes.

Support for the patient

- If it is safe to do so, let the patient know that you are making the social care referral. You are able to make a social care referral without the patient's consent in the interests of child safeguarding.
- If a safety plan is needed, ensure there is one in place before the patient leaves.
- Consider referral to other local support services. This can include, but is not limited to, your local CSE services, local counselling services, updating the school, local special educational needs support services if appropriate.
- Plan with the patient about what will happen when they leave you. Do they want help telling a parent or guardian? How will they get home? What about use of their phone and social media?
- Consider seeking support from the NSPCC via its helpline.

 Spotting the Signs of Child Abuse (NSPCC, 2023c).

Trafficking

Trafficking is defined as two of the following having taken place for the purposes of exploitation: recruitment, transportation or harbouring.

Things to consider
- Trafficking does not only take place across the borders of countries. A person can be trafficked from one town or city to another.
- A person can be trafficked for a number of reasons including sexual exploitation, criminal activity, benefit fraud, forced marriage, domestic servitude or forced labour.
- Trafficking in the context of a sexual health consultation is important, as you may have the opportunity to notice that something does not seem right, for example a patient who is not allowed to come into a health appointment alone, someone who does not have access to things like a phone or passport in the way that other patients do, or noticing physical signs during an intimate examination.
- Adults who have been trafficked may be very reluctant to engage with services, as their immigration status might be a factor.

Professional obligations
- If you have concerns that a child is being trafficked, you have no option but to make a social care referral, and if there is an immediate risk call 999.
- Talk to your patient alone if possible.
- If the patient is an adult, do not forget to consider any children that might be involved.
- Alongside the other safeguarding action you are taking, you must report to the Local Slavery Safeguarding Lead and ask for advice.

Support
- Your organisation, or the local authority, may have a Human Trafficking Champion you can seek advice from.
- Call the Modern Slavery Helpline or get into contact via its website. You can speak to a trained advisor, who is able to give you specific advice and may arrange to speak to your patient. You can speak to them confidentially if you do not know what to do next.

■ Taking a Safeguarding History

You cannot take a good sexual health history without taking a good safeguarding history, and vice versa. When patients come to speak to an HCP about their contraception and sexual health, they are asking for help which, by the very reason for their attendance, is more intimate. This puts us in a unique position to make a holistic assessment and offer help. The same principles of building a good rapport, ensuring that you are non-judgemental and therefore can ask questions that other HCPs may shy away from, and being open and honest with your patient, underpin both. Table 8.6 lists some principles and tips that may help.

Table 8.6 Principles and tips for taking a good safeguarding history.

Principles of safeguarding history taking	Practical tips
Be honest and upfront with the patient.	Consider explaining the limits of confidentiality at the beginning of each consultation, for example: 'What you tell me is confidential, but if you let me know something that makes me worry about you, or someone else, particularly a child, then we may need to make a plan about that before you leave'.
Speak to all patients alone if possible.	Regardless of their age, and even if it is only for part of the consultation. You may find it easier to do this at the beginning of the consultation, as it can be harder to get a support worker, family member, friend or partner to leave mid-way through. Alternatively, explain at the beginning that it is best practice to speak to patients alone, early in the consultation.
Ask open questions.	This can be particularly difficult if you are already busy, running late or feeling stressed. We can close patients down by asking closed questions. Examples of closed questions include: 'Are you OK?' or 'Is that all then?'. If you are worried, you are more likely to elicit information by asking 'Can you tell me more about that?' or 'Is there something else you would like to discuss?'.
If you are starting out, do not worry about having to use a crib sheet.	It can be difficult to remember everything. Consider using some guidance, for example the NSPCC's 'Spotting the Signs' (NSPCC, 2023c). You may also find more information on the BASHH website or on your local authority website.
If you are worried, then try to leave the consultation and get advice immediately.	If there is a safeguarding lead in your organisation that you can talk to there and then, you may find this easier than trying to contact the patient later – particularly if you have concerns that might need urgent action. This will also give you an opportunity to consider what the patient has told you, without being swayed by what actions they want you to take or not to take.
Explain to the patient that you will call them back if anything comes to mind.	If this is likely to be from a withheld number, then also tell the patient this.

CHAPTER 8 • Safeguarding

Table 8.6 (Continued)

Principles of safeguarding history taking	Practical tips
If you ask the patient to come back, ensure they know what will happen if they do not.	For example, if you want to see a patient for a follow-up appointment, as this will give you time to formulate a plan, or you need further information from the patient and you are already running late, then ensure they know that if they do not attend, you may need to share information without speaking to them. This will mean that you can tell social care that the patient was aware that information would be shared without their consent.
If you do not have up-to-date details from the patient, including the details of any relevant others, for example, their partner, children, others they may be caring for, then ask.	It is very difficult to make a social care referral without the correct patient details. It might be possible for social care, or the NHS, to find out who a child is if you have the mother's details, but it is nearly impossible to do the same if you only have the father's details. It can also be very time-consuming.
Be accurate in your record keeping.	There is more information about this below.
Believe what your patient is telling you.	You need to ask questions in order to give good-quality patient care and to make appropriate referrals. It is not our job to investigate or judge.

■ Documentation

Accurate and up-to-date documentation of safeguarding concerns is vital so that patterns are recognised at an early stage and the correct referrals can be put in place. Here are some top tips on documentation when considering safeguarding.

- Only write facts, not opinions or value judgements; for example, 'The patient was crying' not 'The patient did not seem upset enough'.
- Make direct quotes clear; for example, 'The patient stated "They hit me on the face"'.
- Ensure that all records are stored according to your organisation's policies and guidance.
- If you needed more detailed information, write down any leading questions you needed to ask; for example, 'The patient was crying, and so I asked…'.

- Be aware that a patient can ask to see their records.
- Be aware that your notes may be called to court or another member of staff may need to write a report based on your notes.

■ Looking After Yourself

Safeguarding work is hard. It is important to ensure that you have proper support and supervision in place in order to carry out this work safely and effectively. One of the things that makes this work particularly difficult is that you may be dealing with circumstances that are upsetting and confidential. You may not want to bring these circumstances into your home or personal life and offload. For example, if you explain to a loved one that you have had a bad day because you have been working with a patient with cancer, it is easy for everyone to understand why that will have been stressful. It can be more difficult to have the same conversations about safeguarding, particularly with something emotive like a sexual abuse case, for example.

Try to ensure that:

- you have a trusted colleague in work that you can offload to
- you have support strategies in place, for example, spending time outside, going to a class, meeting with friends, counselling or therapy
- if a patient is still on your mind a couple of days after seeing them, talk to someone at work again
- you are kind to yourself. Acknowledge the good work you have done on behalf of this patient, even if the patient does not see that for themselves. Allow yourself to have feelings about this episode of care and try to acknowledge them in a safe space. Be aware that there is a whole process alongside and behind you. It is not your responsibility to do this work alone
- you have supervision if possible.

CASE STUDY

Presenting complaint

Harper, a 32-year-old woman, comes to clinic with symptoms of a UTI.

History

History of presenting complaint

You notice that Harper attends every 2–3 months with vague, low-level symptoms.

CHAPTER 8 • Safeguarding

Past medical/family/drug history
- Harper is married with two children: Sophia, who is 10 years old, and Callum, who is seven years old.
- On further discussion, Harper tells you she is worried her partner is having other sexual partners and things are not good at home. You ask Harper an open question to elicit more information, and she tells you that the children are often upset when her partner comes home.
- You ask her if they have experienced abuse or violence at home, and Harper starts to cry. She tells you that the arguments have become more and more violent, and that recently Harper was hit by her partner, whilst the children were asleep upstairs.
- You ask Harper if there has ever been any sexual abuse, and Harper denies this.

Examination
- Carry out investigations for a UTI.
- Complete a full sexual health screen.
- Ask Harper if she has any injuries, review them and document them in your notes.

Management plan
- Explain to Harper that you believe what she is telling you, and you are concerned about her and the children.
- Complete an assessment with Harper, asking more questions about:
  - the most recent episode, and exactly what happened
  - the frequency of the arguments, abuse or violence
  - exactly where the children have been during these episodes
  - if Harper has any support at the moment.
- Explain to Harper what support is available.
  - IDSVAs and services.
  - A social care referral to ensure that the children have all the support they need.
  - Liaison with the school to support the children.
- You make a safety plan with Harper.
  - You agree that Harper is not able to go home this evening, and she will go to a trusted friend's with her children.
  - You talk about what Harper will say if her partner calls.
  - You advise Harper to make contact with the police.
  - Harper agrees to make contact with the IDSVA before leaving the clinic.
- Whilst Harper is calling the IDSVA, you speak to your safeguarding lead for support.

- You agree a follow-up plan with Harper.
  - Text results for her tests.
  - A follow-up appointment in two weeks' time.
  - An emergency plan if her partner gets in touch – Harper will call the police, make sure she is in a safe space, not answer the door if she is indoors.
- After Harper leaves the clinic you:
  - review your contemporaneous notes
  - make your children's social care referral, ensuring you document your concerns from the children's perspective
  - contact the children's school.
- Make a note on the children's practice records.

References

Adults with Incapacity (Scotland) Act 2000 (asp 4). Available at: https://www.legislation.gov.uk/asp/2000/4/contents [accessed 18 August 2023].

Allen-Leap M et al. (2022). Seeking help from primary health-care providers in high-income countries: a scoping review of the experiences of migrant and refugee survivors of domestic violence. *Trauma Violence Abuse*, 24(5): 3715–3731.

Annon J (1976). The PLISSIT model: a proposed conceptual scheme for the behavioural treatment of sexual problems. *Journal of Sex Education and Therapy*, 2(1): 1–15.

Ashby J et al. (2021). *BASHH National Guideline on the Management of Sexually Transmitted Infections and Related Conditions in Children and Young People*. Available at: https://www.bashhguidelines.org/media/1262/children-and-yp-2021.pdf [accessed 18 August 2023].

Association for Young People's Health (AYPH) (2021). *Key Data on Young People, 2021*. Available at: https://ayph-youthhealthdata.org.uk/key-data/ [accessed 19 December 2023].

Bauer M, Haesler E and Fetherstonhaugh D (2016). Let's talk about sex: older people's views on the recognition of sexuality and sexual health in the health-care setting. *Health Expectations*, 19(6): 1237–1250.

Best O (2017). The cultural safety journey: An Aboriginal Australian nursing and midwifery context. In: Best O and Fredericks B (eds) *Yatdjuligin: Aboriginal and Torres Strait Islander Nursing and Midwifery Care*. Cambridge: Cambridge University Press: 46–66.

Bharadwaj P et al. (2011). What influences young women to choose between the emergency contraceptive pill and an intrauterine device? A qualitative study. *European Journal of Reproductive Healthcare*, 16(3): 201–209.

Brady M et al. (2019). BHIVA/BASHH guidelines on the use of HIV pre-exposure prophylaxis (PrEP) 2018. *HIV Medicine*, 20 Suppl 2: s2–s80.

British Association for Sexual Health and HIV (BASHH) (2019a). *BASHH Recommendations for Integrated Sexual Health Services for Trans, Including Non-Binary, People.* Available at: https://www.bashh.org/about-bashh/publications/ [accessed 30 August 2023].

British Association for Sexual Health and HIV (BASHH) (2019b). *PID.* Available at: https://www.bashhguidelines.org/current-guidelines/systemic-presentation-and-complications/pid-2019/ [accessed 4 July 2022].

British Association for Sexual Health and HIV (BASHH) (2021). *Guidelines.* Available at: https://www.bashh.org/guidelines [accessed 12 December 2023].

British HIV Association (BHIVA) (2020). *BHIVA/BASHH/BIA Adult HIV Testing Guidelines 2020.* Available at: https://www.bhiva.org/HIV-testing-guidelines [accessed 18 August 2023].

British HIV Association/British Association for Sexual Health and HIV (BHIVA/BASHH) (2018). *BHIVA/BASHH Guidelines on the Use of HIV Pre-exposure Prophylaxis (PrEP).* Available at: https://www.bhiva.org/file/5b729cd592060/2018-PrEP-Guidelines.pdf [accessed 17 August 2023].

British Menopause Society (BMS) (2020). *British Menopause Society Fact Sheet: A woman's relationship with the menopause is complicated...* Available at: https://www.womens-health-concern.org/wp-content/uploads/2020/09/BMS-Infographic-A-womans-relationship-with-the-menopause-SEPT2020.jpg [accessed 19 December 2023].

British Menopause Society (BMS) (2020). *BMS Vision for Menopause Care.* Available at: https://thebms.org.uk/publications/bms-vision/ [accessed 30 May 2022].

British Menopause Society (BMS) (2022). *Understanding the Risks of Breast Cancer.* Available at: https://thebms.org.uk/wp-content/uploads/2023/01/WHC-Infographics-JANUARY-2023-BreastCancerRisks.pdf [accessed 4 September 2023].

British Menopause Society (BMS) (2023). *Principles and Practice of Menopause Care.* Available at: https://thebms.org.uk/education/principles-practice-of-menopause-care/ [accessed 26 September 2023].

British Society for Sexual Medicine (2023). *Position Statement for Management of Genitourinary Syndrome of the Menopause.* Available at: https://bssm.org.uk/wp-content/uploads/2023/02/GSM-BSSM.pdf [accessed 14 September 2023].

Brook G et al. (2020). UK National Guideline for consultations requiring sexual history taking: Clinical Effectiveness Group British Association for Sexual Health and HIV. *International Journal of STD and AIDS,* 31(10): 920–928.

Care Act 2014 (c. 23). Available at: https://www.legislation.gov.uk/ukpga/2014/23/contents/enacted [accessed 18 August 2023].

Change Grow Live (2022). *What is Chemsex? Support, Advice and How To Stay Safe.* Available at: https://www.changegrowlive.org/advice-info/alcohol-drugs/chemsex-drugs [accessed 17 August 2023].

References

Children Act 2004 (c. 31). Available at: https://www.legislation.gov.uk/ukpga/2004/31/contents [accessed 8 December 2023].

Children's Society (2021). *Children, Young People and Modern Slavery: A guide for professionals*. Available at: https://www.teescpp.org.uk/media/1328/cyp-and-modern-slavery-final-version.pdf [accessed 18 August 2023].

Coudray M and Madhivanan P (2019). Bacterial vaginosis: a brief synopsis of the literature. *European Journal of Obstetrics and Gynaecology and Reproductive Biology*, 245: 143–148.

Daisy Network (2023). *What is POI?* Available at: https://www.daisynetwork.org/about-poi/what-is-poi/ [accessed 17 August 2023].

Dennerstein GJ et al. (2018). Depot medroxyprogesterone acetate and bone mineral density. *Journal of Clinical Gynaecology and Obstetrics*, 7(3): 63–68.

Ezhova I et al. (2020). Barriers to older adults seeking sexual health advice and treatment: a scoping review. *International Journal of Nursing Studies*, 107: 103566.

Faculty of Sexual and Reproductive Healthcare (FSRH) (2015). *Problematic Bleeding with Hormonal Contraception*. Available at: https://www.fsrh.org/standards-and-guidance/documents/ceuguidanceproblematicbleedinghormonalcontraception/ [accessed 30 August 2023].

Faculty of Sexual and Reproductive Healthcare (FSRH) (2016). *UK Medical Eligibility Criteria*. Available at: https://www.fsrh.org/ukmec/ [accessed 12 December 2023].

Faculty of Sexual and Reproductive Healthcare (FSRH) (2017). *Contraceptive Choices and Sexual Health for Transgender and Non-Binary People*. Available at: https://www.fsrh.org/documents/fsrh-ceu-statement-contraceptive-choices-and-sexual-health-for/ [accessed 14 August 2023].

Faculty of Sexual and Reproductive Healthcare (FSRH) (2018). *RCGP Menstrual Wellbeing Toolkit for Use by GPs*. Available at: https://www.fsrh.org/news/rcgp-creates-menstrual-wellbeing-toolkit-for-use-by-gps/ [accessed 18 April 2022].

Faculty of Sexual and Reproductive Healthcare (FSRH) (2019a). *Clinical Guideline: Contraception for women aged over 40 years*. Available at: https://www.fsrh.org/documents/fsrh-guidance-contraception-for-women-aged-over-40-years-2017/ [accessed 30 August 2023].

Faculty of Sexual and Reproductive Healthcare (FSRH) (2019b). *Overweight, Obesity and Contraception*. Available at: https://www.fsrh.org/standards-and-guidance/documents/fsrh-clinical-guideline-overweight-obesity-and-contraception/ [accessed 14 August 2023].

Faculty of Sexual and Reproductive Healthcare (FSRH) (2019c). *FSRH CEU Statement on Antibiotic Cover for Urgent Insertion of Intrauterine Contraception in Women at High Risk of STI*. Available at: https://www.fsrh.org/standards-and-guidance/documents/fsrh-ceu-statement-on-antibiotic-cover-for-urgent-insertion-of/ [accessed 4 July 2022].

Faculty of Sexual and Reproductive Healthcare (FSRH) (2020a). *FSRH Clinical Guidelines: Contraception after pregnancy*. Available at: https://www.fsrh.org/documents/contraception-after-pregnancy-guideline-january-2017/ [accessed 14 August 2023].

Faculty of Sexual and Reproductive Healthcare (FSRH) (2020b). *FSRH Clinical Guideline: Emergency contraception*. Available at: https://www.fsrh.org/standards-and-guidance/documents/ceu-clinical-guidance-emergency-contraception-march-2017/ [accessed 12 December 2023].

Faculty of Sexual and Reproductive Healthcare (FSRH) (2021). *FSRH Statement: Pain Associated with Insertion of Intrauterine Contraception*. Available at: https://www.fsrh.org/standards-and-guidance/documents/fsrh-statement-pain-associated-with-insertion-of-intrauterine/ [accessed 2 January 2024].

Faculty of Sexual and Reproductive Healthcare (FSRH) (2023a). *Intrauterine Contraception*. Available at: https://www.fsrh.org/standards-and-guidance/documents/ceuguidanceintrauterinecontraception/ [accessed 14 August 2023].

Faculty of Sexual and Reproductive Healthcare (FSRH) (2023b). *Combined Hormonal Contraception*. Available at: https://www.fsrh.org/standards-and-guidance/documents/combined-hormonal-contraception/ [accessed 14 August 2023].

Faculty of Sexual and Reproductive Health (FSRH) (2023c). *Essentials of Menopause Care*. Available at: https://www.fsrh.org/education-and-training/essentials-of-menopause-care/ [accessed 19 December 2023].

Faculty of Sexual and Reproductive Health (FSRH) (2024). *FSRH CEU Statement: Mirena 8 years contraception*. Available at: https://www.fsrh.org/documents/fsrh-ceu-statement-mirena-8-years-contraception-jan-2024/#:~:text=The%20United%20Kingdom%20Medicines%20Health,to%208%20years%20for%20contraception. [accessed 19 January 2024].

Family Planning Association (FPA) (2020). *Your Guide to Contraception*. Available at: https://www.fpa.org.uk/download/your-guide-to-contraception/ [accessed 14 August 2023].

Gore-Gorszewska G (2020). "Why not ask the doctor?" Barriers in help-seeking for sexual problems among older adults in Poland. *International Journal of Public Health*, 65(8): 1507–1515.

Gov.UK (2021). *Statement Opposing FGM leaflet*. Available at: https://www.gov.uk/government/publications/statement-opposing-female-genital-mutilation [accessed 8 May 2022].

GP Notebook (2021). *Physiological (Normal) Vaginal Discharge*. Available at: https://gpnotebook.com/en-gb/simplepage.cfm?ID=x20130127160448685340 [accessed 30 August 2023].

Griffith R (2016). What is Gillick competence? *Human Vaccines and Immunotherapeutics*, 12(1): 244–247.

References

Hamoda H et al. (2016). The British Menopause Society & Women's Health Concern recommendations on hormone replacement therapy in menopausal women. *Post Reproductive Health*, 22(4): 165–183.

Hashim MS et al. (2019). Premenstrual syndrome is associated with dietary and lifestyle behaviors among university students: a cross-sectional study. *Nutrients*, 11(8): 1939.

Health and Care Professions Council (HCPC) (2016). *Standards of Performance, Conduct and Ethics*. Available at: https://www.hcpc-uk.org/standards/standards-of-conduct-performance-and-ethics/ [accessed 18 August 2023].

Hillard T et al. (2021). *Management of the Menopause*, 6th edn. London: British Menopause Society.

Hinchliff S and Gott M (2011). Seeking medical help for sexual concerns in mid- and later life: a review of the literature. *Journal of Sex Research*, 48(2-3): 106–117.

HIV Lens (2023). Welcome to HIV lens. Available at: https://www.hiv-lens.org/ [accessed 8 December 2023].

HM Government (2018). *Working Together to Safeguard Children: A guide to inter-agency working to safeguard and promote the welfare of children*. Available at: https://www.gov.uk/government/publications/working-together-to-safeguard-children–2 [accessed 8 January 2023].

Home Office (2012). *New Definition of Domestic Violence*. Available at: https://www.gov.uk/government/news/new-definition-of-domestic-violence [accessed 18 August 2023].

Joint Formulary Committee (2023a). Emergency Contraception. *British National Formulary*. Available at: https://bnf.nice.org.uk/treatment-summaries/emergency-contraception/ [accessed 14 August 2023].

Joint Formulary Committee (2023b). Levonorgestrel. *British National Formulary*. Available at: https://bnf.nice.org.uk/drugs/levonorgestrel/#breastfeeding [accessed 12 December 2023].

Lania A et al. (2019). Functional hypothalamic and drug-induced amenorrhea: an overview. *Journal of Endocrinological Investigation*, 42(9): 1001–1010.

Leslie SW, Sajjad H and Kumar S (2023). *Genital Warts [Internet]*. Treasure Island: StatPearls Publishing. Available from: https://www.ncbi.nlm.nih.gov/books/NBK441884/.

Lokugamage AU et al. (2023). Translating Cultural Safety to the UK. *Journal of Medical Ethics*, 49(4): 244–251.

Luby R (2018). *Supporting Patients Who Make Disclosures of Sexual Violence on Inpatient Wards: A practical guide for mental health professionals*. Available at: https://www.rcn.org.uk/-/media/royal-college-of-nursing/documents/clinical-topics/mental-health/rachel-luby-disclosures-of-sexual-violence.pdf?la=en&hash=795ED5602DE53E7F21A22B215B696EED [accessed 14 August 2023].

Mason R (2020). *Emergency Contraception Counselling – OSCE Guide Geeky Medics*. Available at: https://geekymedics.com/emergency-contraception-counselling-osce-guide/ [accessed 12 December 2023].

McCall H et al. (2015). What is chemsex and why does it matter? *BMJ*, 351: h5790.

Menopause Charity (2021). *Rebranding the Menopause as a Female Hormone Deficiency*. Available at: https://www.themenopausecharity.org/2021/05/05/rebranding-the-menopause-as-a-female-hormone-deficiency/ [accessed 22 April 2022].

Menopause matters (2023). *Menopause matters*. Available at: https://www.menopausematters.co.uk/ [accessed 18 December 2023].

Mental Capacity Act 2005 (c. 9). Available at: https://www.legislation.gov.uk/ukpga/2005/9/contents [accessed 18 August 2023].

Mental Capacity Act (Northern Ireland) 2016 (c. 18). Available at: https://www.legislation.gov.uk/nia/2016/18/contents/enacted [accessed 4 September 2023].

Nash P et al. (2015). Sexual health and sexual activity in later life. *Reviews in Clinical Gerontology*, 25(1): 22–30.

National Aids Trust (2021). *Do I understand HIV?* Available at: https://www.nat.org.uk/about-hiv/understanding-hiv [accessed 6 January 2023].

National Health Service (NHS) (2018a). *Trichomoniasis*. Available at: https://www.nhs.uk/conditions/trichomoniasis/ [accessed 12 December 2023].

National Health Service (NHS) (2018b). *Sexual and Reproductive Health Services England*. Available at: https://digital.nhs.uk/data-and-information/publications/statistical/sexual-and-reproductive-health-services/2017-18 [accessed 12 December 2023].

National Health Service (NHS) (2019). *What Should I Do If I Miss a Pill (Combined Pill)?* Available at: https://www.nhs.uk/conditions/contraception/miss-combined-pill/ [accessed 14 August 2023].

National Health Service (NHS) (2020a). *Condoms*. Available at: https://www.nhs.uk/conditions/contraception/male-condoms/ [accessed 14 August 2023].

National Health Service (NHS) (2020b). *Genital Warts*. Available at: https://www.nhs.uk/conditions/genital-warts/ [accessed 12 December 2023].

National Health Service (NHS) (2021a). *The Progestogen Only Pill*. Available at: https://www.nhs.uk/conditions/contraception/the-pill-progestogen-only/ [accessed 14 August 2023].

National Health Service (NHS) (2021b). *Contraceptive Patch*. Available at: https://www.nhs.uk/conditions/contraception/contraceptive-patch/ [accessed 14 August 2023].

National Health Service (NHS) (2021c). *Vaginal Ring*. Available at: https://www.nhs.uk/conditions/contraception/vaginal-ring/ [accessed 14 August 2023].

National Health Service (NHS) (2021d). *Female Condoms*. Available at: https://www.nhs.uk/conditions/contraception/female-condoms/ [accessed 12 December 2023].

References

National Health Service (NHS) (2021e). *Trichomoniasis*. Available at: https://www.nhs.uk/conditions/trichomoniasis/ [accessed 2 January 2024].

National Health Service (NHS) (2022c). *Female Genital Mutilation (FGM)*. Available at: https://www.nhs.uk/conditions/female-genital-mutilation-fgm/ [accessed 18 August 2023].

National Institute for Health and Care Excellence (NICE) (2016). *Contraception*. Available at: https://www.nice.org.uk/guidance/qs129/chapter/quality-statement-4-contraception-after-childbirth [accessed 14 August 2023].

National Institute for Health and Care Excellence (NICE) (2018a). *How Should I Assess for a Secondary Cause of Dysmenorrhoea?* Available at: https://cks.nice.org.uk/topics/dysmenorrhoea/diagnosis/assessment/ [accessed 20 April 2022].

National Institute for Health and Care Excellence (NICE) (2018b). *Menorrhagia (Heavy Menstrual Bleeding)*. Available at: https://cks.nice.org.uk/topics/menorrhagia-heavy-menstrual-bleeding/ [accessed 20 April 2022].

National Institute for Health and Care Excellence (NICE) (2018c). *Bacterial Vaginosis in Women Who are Not Pregnant*. Available at: https://cks.nice.org.uk/topics/bacterial-vaginosis/management/women-who-are-not-pregnant/ [accessed 30 August 2023].

National Institute for Health and Care Excellence (NICE) (2019a). *Management of Premenstrual Syndrome*. Available at: https://cks.nice.org.uk/topics/premenstrual-syndrome/management/management/ [accessed 20 April 2022].

National Institute for Health and Care Excellence (NICE) (2019b). *Menopause: Diagnosis and Management*. Available at: https://www.nice.org.uk/guidance/ng23/chapter/Recommendations [accessed 10 April 2022].

National Institute for Health and Care Excellence (NICE) (2019c). *Management of Suspected Syphilis*. Available at: https://cks.nice.org.uk/topics/syphilis/management/management-of-suspected-syphilis/ [accessed 12 December 2023].

National Institute for Health and Care Excellence (NICE) (2020). *Gonorrhoea*. Available at: https://cks.nice.org.uk/topics/gonorrhoea/ [accessed 12 December 2023].

National Institute for Health and Care Excellence (NICE) (2021a). *Clinical Knowledge Summary: Symptoms suggestive of gynaecological cancers*. Available at: https://cks.nice.org.uk/topics/gynaecological-cancers-recognition-referral/diagnosis/symptoms-suggestive-of-gynaecological-cancers/ [accessed 30 August 2023].

National Institute for Health and Care Excellence (NICE) (2021b). *Management of Uncomplicated Genital Chlamydia*. Available at: https://cks.nice.org.uk/topics/chlamydia-uncomplicated-genital/management/management/ [accessed 8 May 2021].

National Institute for Health and Care Excellence (NICE) (2021c). *Managing Hepatitis B Infection*. Available at: https://cks.nice.org.uk/topics/hepatitis-b/management/managing-hepatitis-b-infection/ [accessed 30 June 2021].

National Institute for Health and Care Excellence (NICE) (2021d). *HIV Infection and AIDS.* https://cks.nice.org.uk/topics/hiv-infection-aids/ [accessed 30 June 2021].

National Institute for Health and Care Excellence (NICE) (2022a). *Reducing Sexually Transmitted Infections.* Available at: https://www.nice.org.uk/guidance/ng221/chapter/Rationale-and-impact [accessed 2 January 2024].

National Institute for Health and Care Excellence (NICE) (2022b). *Amenorrhoea.* Available at: https://cks.nice.org.uk/topics/amenorrhoea/ [accessed 20 April 2022].

National Institute for Health and Care Excellence (NICE) (2022c). *Menopause.* Available at: https://cks.nice.org.uk/topics/menopause/ [accessed 18 August 2023].

National Institute for Health and Care Excellence (NICE) (2022d). *Hormone Replacement Therapy (HRT).* Available at: https://cks.nice.org.uk/topics/menopause/prescribing-information/hormone-replacement-therapy-hrt/ [accessed 30 August 2023].

National Institute for Health and Care Excellence (NICE) (2022e). *Gonorrhoea.* Available at: https://cks.nice.org.uk/topics/gonorrhoea/ [accessed 21 May 2022].

National Institute for Health and Care Excellence (NICE) (2023). *Herpes Simplex – Genital.* Available at: https://cks.nice.org.uk/topics/herpes-simplex-genital/ [accessed 2 January 2024].

National Society for the Prevention of Cruelty to Children (NSPCC) (2022). *Gillick Competency and Fraser Guidelines*. Available at: https://learning.nspcc.org.uk/child-protection-system/gillick-competence-fraser-guidelines [accessed 18 August 2023].

National Society for the Prevention of Cruelty to Children (NSPCC) (2023a). *Female Genital Mutilation (FGM).* Available at: https://www.nspcc.org.uk/what-is-child-abuse/types-of-abuse/female-genital-mutilation-fgm/ [accessed 8 August 2023].

National Society for the Prevention of Cruelty to Children (NSPCC) (2023b). *Child Sexual Exploitation*. Available at: https://www.nspcc.org.uk/what-is-child-abuse/types-of-abuse/child-sexual-exploitation/ [accessed 18 August 2023].

National Society for the Prevention of Cruelty to Children (NSPCC) (2023c). *Spotting the Signs of Child Abuse.* Available at: https://www.nspcc.org.uk/what-is-child-abuse/spotting-signs-child-abuse/ [accessed 18 August 2023].

Newson Health (2023a). *Balance.* Available at: https://www.balance-menopause.com/ [accessed 18 December 2023].

Newson Health (2023b). *Confidence in the Menopause.* Available at: https://www.newsonhealth.co.uk/confidence-in-the-menopause/ [accessed 18 December 2023].

Newson Health (2023c). *Newson Health Menopause Society.* Available at: https://www.nhmenopausesociety.org/ [accessed 18 December 2023].

Newson L (2021). *Menopause Symptom Questionnaire.* Available at: https://www.balance-menopause.com/menopause-library/menopause-symptom-sheet/ [accessed 30 August 2023].

References

Newson L and Mair R (2018). Results from the BJFM menopause survey. *British Journal of Family Medicine*, 6(1): 12–22.

Nursing and Midwifery Council (2023). *The Code*. Available at: https://www.nmc.org.uk/standards/code/ [accessed 18 August 2023].

Panay N (2018). GSM/VVA: advances in understanding and management. In: Birkhaeuser A and Genazzani AR (eds) *Pre-menopause, Menopause and Beyond. Volume 5: Frontiers in Gynaecological Endocrinology*. Berlin: Springer: 261–268.

Panay N, Briggs P and Kovacs G (2015). *Managing the Menopause: 21st century solutions*. Cambridge: Cambridge University Press.

Parker W (2022). *Menstrual Disorders*. Available at: https://www.healthywomen.org/condition/menstrual-disorders/overview [accessed 20 April 2022].

Pearlstein T and Steiner M (2008). Premenstrual dysphoric disorder: burden of illness and treatment update. *Journal of Psychiatry and Neuroscience*, 33(4): 291–301.

Ports KA et al. (2014). Sexual health discussions with older patients during periodic health exams. *Journal of Sexual Medicine*, 11(4): 901–908.

Public Health England (PHE) (2018). *Teenage Pregnancy Prevention Framework*. Available at: https://www.gov.uk/government/publications/teenage-pregnancy-prevention-framework [accessed 12 December 2023].

Public Health England (PHE) (2019). *Sexually Transmitted Infections and Screening for Chlamydia in England*. Available at: https://assets.publishing.service.gov.uk/government/uploads/system/uploads/attachment_data/file/914249/STI_NCSP_report_2019.pdf [accessed 2 January 2024].

Public Health England (PHE) (2021). *Changes to the National Chlamydia Screening Programme (NCSP)*. Available at: https://assets.publishing.service.gov.uk/media/60d0782ad3bf7f4bd11a2416/NCSP_Public_Sector_Equality_Duty_Assessment_June_2021.pdf [accessed 30 August 2023].

Ramdhan RC, Simonds E and Tubbs SR (2018). Complications of subcutaneous contraceptives: a review. *Cureus*, 10(1): e2132.

Rape Crisis (2023). *What is Sexual Violence?* Available at: https://rapecrisis.org.uk/get-informed/about-sexual-violence/what-is-sexual-violence/ [accessed 18 August 2023].

Rowlands S, Oloto E and Horwell DH (2016). Intrauterine devices and risk of uterine perforation: current perspectives. *Open Access Journal of Contraception*, 7: 19–32.

Sexual Offences Act 2003 (c. 42). Available at: https://www.legislation.gov.uk/ukpga/2003/42/contents [accessed 18 August 2023].

Sexwise (2021). *Let's Talk About Sex!* Available at: https://www.sexwise.org.uk/ [accessed 12 December 2023].

Shaw I (2020). *Menopause – Guidance on management and prescribing HRT for GPs*. Available at: https://pcwhf.co.uk/wp-content/uploads/2023/02/Prescribing-HRT.pdf [accessed 18 December 2023].

Simmons KB et al. (2018). Drug interactions between rifamycin antibiotics and hormonal contraception: a systematic review. *British Journal of Obstetrics and Gynaecology*, 125(7): 804–811.

Taylor B and Davis S (2007). The Extended PLISSIT Model for addressing the sexual wellbeing of individuals with an acquired disability or chronic illness. *Sexuality and Disability*, 25: 135–139.

Terrence Higgins Trust (2023). Available at: https://www.tht.org.uk/ [accessed 30 August 2023].

Tiwari K, Khanam I and Savarna N (2018). A study on effectiveness of lactational amenorrhea as a method of contraception. *International Journal of Reproduction, Contraception, Obstetrics and Gynaecology*, 7(10): 3946–3950.

UK Health Security Agency (2023). *Annual Epidemiological Spotlight on HIV in London: 2021 data*. Available at: https://www.gov.uk/government/publications/hiv-london-annual-data-spotlight/annual-epidemiological-spotlight-on-hiv-in-london-2021-data [accessed 14 September 2023].

Wightman Lawson G (2021). Naegele's rule and the length of pregnancy – a review. *Australian and New Zealand Journal of Obstetrics and* Gynaecology, 61(2): 177–182.

Women's Health Concern (2023). *For patients*. Available at: https://www.womens-health-concern.org/ [accessed 18 December 2023].

Women's Health Initiative (WHI) (2002). Risks and benefits of estrogen plus progestin in healthy postmenopausal women: principal results from the Women's Health Initiative randomized controlled trial. *Journal of the American Medical Association*, 288(3): 321–333.

World Health Organization (WHO) (2017). *Global Hepatitis Report, 2017*. Available at: https://apps.who.int/iris/bitstream/handle/10665/255016/9789241565455-eng.pdf [accessed 14 September 2023].

World Health Organization (WHO) (2022). *Female Genital Mutilation*. Available at: https://www.who.int/news-room/fact-sheets/detail/female-genital-mutilation [accessed 18 August 2023].

Further Reading

British Association for Sexual Health and HIV (BASHH) (2014). Available at: https://portal.e-lfh.org.uk/AICC_Content/GUM_01_012/d/ELFH_Session_4_20/588/resources.html [accessed 2 January 2024].

British Association for Sexual Health and HIV (BASHH) (2022). *BASHH Guidelines*. Available at: https://www.bashh.org/guidelines [accessed 17 August 2023].

British Association of Urological Surgeons (2023). *Patients: I think I might have...* Available at: https://www.baus.org.uk/patients/conditions/ [accessed 4 September 2023].

British HIV Association/British Association for Sexual Health and HIV/British Infection Association (BHIVA/BASHH/BIA) (2020). *Adult HIV Testing Guidelines 2020*. Available at: https://www.bhiva.org/file/5f68c0dd7aefb/HIV-testing-guidelines-2020.pdf [accessed 17 August 2023].

BritSPAG (2019). *What is a Vulva Anyway?* Available at: https://britspag.org/wp-content/uploads/2019/06/So_what_is_a_vulva_anyway_final_booklet.pdf [accessed 17 August 2023].

Brook G et al. (2020). UK National Guideline for consultations requiring sexual history taking: Clinical Effectiveness Group British Association for Sexual Health and HIV. *International Journal of STD and AIDS*, 31(10): 920–928.

Campbell C (2015). *The Relate Guide to Sexual Intimacy*. London: Vermillion.

Care Quality Commission (2022). *GP Mythbuster 8: Gillick Competency and Fraser Guidelines*. Available at: https://www.cqc.org.uk/guidance-providers/gps/gp-mythbusters/gp-mythbuster-8-gillick-competency-fraser-guidelines#:~:text=Gillick%20competence%20is%20concerned%20with,sexual%20health%20advice%20and%20treatment [accessed 18 August 2023].

Centers for Disease Control and Prevention (CDC) (2019). *Discussing Sexual Health with Your Patients*. Available at: https://www.cdc.gov/hiv/pdf/clinicians/screening/cdc-hiv-php-discussing-sexual-health.pdf [accessed 17 August 2023].

Change Grow Live (2022). Available at: https://www.changegrowlive.org/ [accessed 17 August 2023].

The Clare Project (2021). *Supporting Transgender Adults: a guide for primary care practitioners*. Available at: https://clareproject.org.uk/wp-content/uploads/2021/09/TCP_Resource-for-GPs.pdf [accessed 4 September 2023].

Daisy Network (2023). *What is POI?* Available at: https://www.daisynetwork.org/ [accessed 17 August 2023]

Department of Health (2016). *Female Genital Mutilation Risk and Safeguarding: Guidance for professionals*. London: Department of Health. https://assets.publishing.service.gov.uk/government/uploads/system/uploads/attachment_data/file/525390/FGM_safeguarding_report_A.pdf [accessed 17 August 2023].

Faculty of Sexual and Reproductive Health (FSRH) (2010). *FSRH Clinical Guidelines: Contraceptive Choices for Young People*. Available at: https://www.fsrh.org/standards-and-guidance/documents/cec-ceu-guidance-young-people-mar-2010/ [accessed 17 August 2023].

Faculty of Sexual and Reproductive Healthcare (FSRH) (2015). *Problematic Bleeding with Hormonal Contraception*. Available at: https://www.fsrh.org/standards-and-guidance/documents/ceuguidanceproblematicbleedinghormonalcontraception/ [accessed 17 August 2023].

Faculty of Sexual and Reproductive Healthcare (FSRH) (2016). *UK Medical Eligibility Criteria for Contraceptive Use: UKMEC 2016 (Amended September 2019)*. Available at: https://www.fsrh.org/documents/ukmec-2016/ [accessed 17 August 2023].

Faculty of Sexual and Reproductive Health (FSRH) (2020a). *FSRH Clinical Guideline: Contraception After Pregnancy*. Available at: https://www.fsrh.org/standards-and-guidance/documents/contraception-after-pregnancy-guideline-january-2017/ [accessed 14 August 2023].

Faculty of Sexual and Reproductive Health (FSRH) (2020b). *FSRH Clinical Guideline: Emergency Contraception*. Available at: https://www.fsrh.org/documents/ceu-clinical-guidance-emergency-contraception-march-2017/ [accessed 17 August 2023].

Herpes Virus Association (2022). Available at: https://herpes.org.uk/ [accessed 17 August 2023].

Home Office (2018). *Domestic Abuse: How to get help*. Available at: https://www.gov.uk/guidance/domestic-abuse-how-to-get-help [accessed 18 August 2023].

McCartney J (2022). *The Great Wall of Vulva*. Available at: https://www.thegreatwallofvulva.com/ [accessed 17 August 2023].

National Health Service (NHS) (2019). *What Should I Do If I Miss a Pill (Combined Pill)?* Available at: https://www.nhs.uk/conditions/contraception/miss-combined-pill/ [accessed 14 August 2023].

Further Reading

National Health Service (NHS) (2021a). *The Progestogen Only Pill*. Available at: https://www.nhs.uk/conditions/contraception/the-pill-progestogen-only/ [accessed 12 December 2023].

National Health Service (NHS) (2021b). *Contraceptive Patch*. Available at: https://www.nhs.uk/conditions/contraception/contraceptive-patch/ [accessed 14 August 2023].

National Health Service (NHS) (2021c). *Vaginal Ring*. Available at: https://www.nhs.uk/conditions/contraception/vaginal-ring/ [accessed 12 December 2023].

National Health Service (NHS) (2021e). *Vaginal Discharge*. Available at: https://www.nhs.uk/conditions/vaginal-discharge/ [accessed 22 August 2023].

National Health Service (NHS) (2022b). *Benefits and Risks of Hormone Replacement Therapy (HRT)*. Available at: https://www.nhs.uk/conditions/hormone-replacement-therapy-hrt/risks/ [accessed 22 August 2023].

National Health Service (NHS) (2023). *Men's Health*. Available at: https://www.nhs.uk/common-health-questions/mens-health/ [accessed 22 August 2023].

National Health Service (NHS) England (2022a). *Chaperones and consent*. Available at: https://www.gmc-uk.org/professional-standards/professional-standards-for-doctors/intimate-examinations-and-chaperones/intimate-examinations-and-chaperones [accessed 2 January 2024].

National Institute for Health and Care Excellence (NICE) (2021b). *Gynaecological Cancers – Recognition and Referral*. Available at: https://cks.nice.org.uk/topics/gynaecological-cancers-recognition-referral/ [accessed 18 August 2023].

National Society for the Prevention of Cruelty to Children (NSPCC) Learning (2022). *Gillick Competency and Fraser Guidelines*. Available at: https://learning.nspcc.org.uk/child-protection-system/gillick-competence-fraser-guidelines [accessed 18 August 2023].

National Society for the Prevention of Cruelty to Children (NSPCC) (2023c). *Spotting the Signs of Child Abuse*. Available at: https://www.nspcc.org.uk/what-is-child-abuse/spotting-signs-child-abuse/ [accessed 18 August 2023].

Rape Crisis (2023). *Get Help*. Available at: https://rapecrisis.org.uk/get-help/ [accessed 18 August 2023].

Royal College of General Practitioners Learning (2023). *LGBT Health Hub*. Available at: https://elearning.rcgp.org.uk/course/view.php?id=584 [accessed 2 January 2024].

Sexual Wellbeing for All (2023). *Sexual Wellbeing Resources*. Available at: https://sexualwellbeingforall.wordpress.com [accessed 14 September 2023].

Sexwise (2021). *Combined Pill (COC)*. Available at: https://www.sexwise.org.uk/contraception/combined-pill-coc [accessed 22 August 2023].

Social Care Institute for Excellence (SCIE) (2011). *Think Child, Think Parent, Think Family: A guide to parental mental health and child welfare*. Available at: https://www.scie.org.uk/publications/guides/guide30/introduction/thinkchild.asp [accessed 18 August 2023].

Stephens E et al. (2021). HRT – *Practical prescribing*. Available at: https://thebms.org.uk/wp-content/uploads/2022/03/03-BMS-TfC-HRT-Practical-Prescribing-OCT2021-01B.pdf [accessed 22 August 2023].

TransActual (2021). *Supporting Trans Patients: A quick guide for GPs*. Available at: https://www.transactual.org.uk/gp-support-trans [accessed 4 September 2023].

University of Liverpool (2022). *HIV Drug Interactions*. Available at: https://www.hiv-druginteractions.org/checker [accessed 22 August 2023].

Vincent B (2018). *Transgender Health: A practitioner's guide to binary and non-binary trans patient care*. London: Jessica Kingsley Publishers.

Women's Aid (2022). *Safety Planning*. Available at: https://www.womens-aid.org.uk/saftey-planning [accessed 14 September 2023].

Index

A

Accountability, 105
Adults with Incapacity (Scotland) Act 2000, 107
Amenorrhoea, 55
　causes, 62
　diagnosis, 62
　management, 62–63
Annon, Jack, 5

B

Bacterial vaginosis, 99–100
BMS. *See* British Menopause Society (BMS)
Breast cancer, 79
Breastfeeding, 37
British Association for Sexual Health and HIV (BASHH), 9
British Menopause Society (BMS), 71

C

Candida, 100–101
Cardiovascular risk, 80
Chemsex, 10
Child sexual exploitation, 115–116
Chlamydia, 87–89

Combined oral contraceptive pill (COCP), 28–31
Combined transdermal patch, 31–32
Combined vaginal ring, 32–33
Condoms, 34
Confidentiality, 110–111
Contraception, 19–38
　barrier methods, 34–35
　examination, 21
　health promotion, 37–38
　history, 19–21
　problematic bleeding, 63–64
　transgender and non-binary people, 36–37
　types
　　contraceptive implant, 25–26
　　copper IUD, 27–28
　　intrauterine contraception, 26–27
　　long-acting reversible contraception, 23–25
　　progestogen-only pill, 22–23
Contraceptive implant, 25–26
Copper IUD, 27–28, 45
Cultural safety, 3–4

D

Davis, Sally, 5
Diaphragms, 34–35

137

Index

Domestic violence and abuse, 113–114
Dysmenorrhoea, 55
    causes, 59
    diagnosis, 58
    management, 59–60

E

Emergency contraception (EC)
    and breastfeeding, 52
    comparison, 47–48
    consideration of STIs, 43
    consultation flowchart, 42
    examination, 43
    history, 43
    indications for, 41–42
    methods, 45–46
    pregnancy testing, 52
    safeguarding, 44
    and transgender individuals, 49–52
    use of, 49
Empowerment, 105
Ex-PLISSIT model, 5
External female genitalia, 17
External male genitalia, 18

F

Faculty of Sexual and Reproductive Healthcare (FSRH), 19, 36
Female genital mutilation (FGM), 9, 10, 114–115
Female reproductive system, 13–16
    calculating gestation, pregnancy, 14–15
    contraception and fertility, 15
    menstrual cycle, 14
    vaginal discharge, 15–16
Female sterilisation, 35
FGM. *See* Female genital mutilation (FGM)
Follicle-stimulating hormone testing, 74
Fraser Guidelines, 109–110

G

Genital herpes, 90–92
Genital warts, 92
Gillick Competence, 109
Gonorrhoea, 89–90

H

Health and Care Professions Council (HCPC), 110
Healthcare professionals (HCPs), 1
Health promotion
    breastfeeding, 37
    contraception after childbirth, 37
    opportunities, 37–38
Hepatitis B, 94–95
Hormone replacement therapy, 77–81
    abnormal uterine bleeding in women, 81
    alternative to, 82–83
    benefits and risks of, 78
    prescribing and monitoring, 80–81
Human immunodeficiency virus, 95–98

I

Intrauterine contraception, 26–27

L

Levonorgestrel, 46
Long-acting reversible contraception, 23–25

M

Male fertility, 17
Male reproductive system, 16–17
Menopause
    definition, 73
    diagnosis, 74–76
    information sharing and advice, 76
    introduction, 71–73
    management of, 76–77

resources, 83
symptoms, 73–74
Menorrhagia, 55
  causes, 60
  diagnosis, 60
  management, 61
Menstrual cycle, 14
Menstrual-related complications
  examination, 57–58
  history, 56
  introduction, 55
  types, 55
Mental Capacity Act 2005, 106
Mental Capacity Act (Northern Ireland) 2016, 107–109

N

National Institute for Health and Care Excellence (NICE), 19, 46
National Society for the Prevention of Cruelty to Children (NSPCC), 110
Nursing and Midwifery Council (NMC), 110

P

Partnership, 105
Peri-menopause
  definition, 73
PLISSIT model, 5
PMS. *See* Premenstrual syndrome (PMS)
Pre-exposure prophylaxis (PrEP), 97, 98
Pregnancy
  calculating gestation, 14–15
Premenstrual syndrome (PMS), 55, 65–68
PrEP. *See* Pre-exposure prophylaxis (PrEP)
Prevention, 105
Progestogen-only pill, 22–23
Proportionality, 105
Protection, 105

S

Safeguarding
  concepts in, 105–111

  documentation, 119
  history, 117–119
  introduction, 103–104
  principles of, 104–105
  regional variability, 104
  scenarios related to sexual health, 111–117
Sexual health issues
  communication skills, 2
  communication with specific groups, 9–12
  cultural safety, 3–4
  environmental factors, 2–3
  history, 6–8
  language challenges in communication, 3
  multiple partners, 8
  self-awareness, 1
  sexual difficulties in men, 9
  sexual difficulties in women, 9
Sexually transmitted infections (STIs), 1
  examination, 86
  history, 85–86
Sexual Offences Act 2003, 105–106
Sexual violence, 111–112
Syphilis, 93–94

T

Taylor, Bridget, 5
Think Family, 111
Trafficking, 116–117
Trichomoniasis, 92–93

U

Ulipristal acetate, 45
Unprotected sexual intercourse (UPSI), 41

V

Vasectomy, 35
Venous thromboembolism risk, 79